# The 100 Foods

## Yo  g

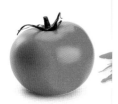

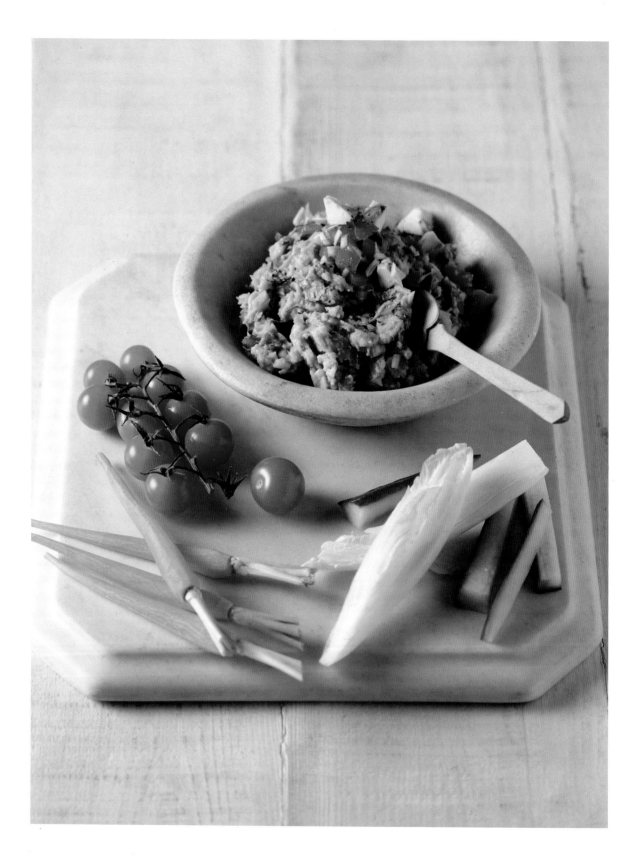

# The 100 Foods
# You Should be Eating

## How to source, prepare and cook healthy ingredients

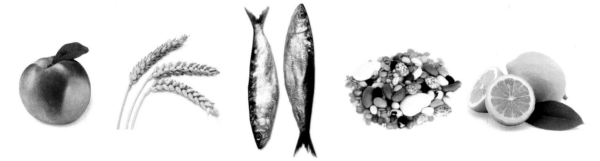

# Glen Matten

NEW
HOLLAND

# Contents

# Introduction

Like many a good idea, the idea behind this book is a simple one. I want you to think differently about the food you put on your plate. That's it. See, I said it was simple. But before you flip the page and rock on with the recipes, here's the lowdown on what this book's all about.

I don't know about you, but when it comes to the food we eat, I reckon I could sum it up in four words: we've lost the plot. I can't imagine there ever being a time when our diets have been the focus of so many TV shows, magazines or news headlines. In fact you can pick up just about any glossy magazine and read about the latest Hollywood diet craze or what your fave celeb is (or more likely isn't) eating. Yet despite all this (so-called) advice we're fatter and less healthy than previous generations. I mean, what's all that about?

I reckon we've forgotten about what's important. Food. The real thing. The stuff nature intended us to eat. Trouble is, we're lost in a world of convenience junk food on the one-hand and shiny vitamin pills and heavily

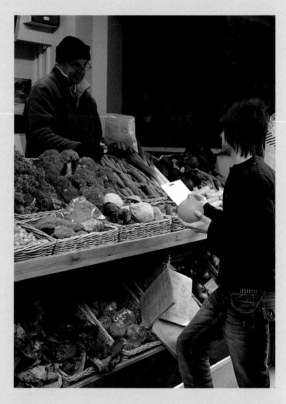

branded 'superfoods' (a bonkers idea if ever there was one) on the other. It's a classic case of not being able to see the wood for the trees. Even if the will is there and you want to make healthy choices, how do you go about making sense of all the marketing gobbledygook and half-truths? And what I really want to know, more than anything else, is how did something that should be so simple get so complicated?

So as far as I'm concerned, it's time to get a few basic things straight. After all, if it's good health you're after, the scientific evidence is pretty clear – eating a healthy diet, including many of the foods featured in this book, is probably one of the best health insurance policies you're likely to take out. And it doesn't

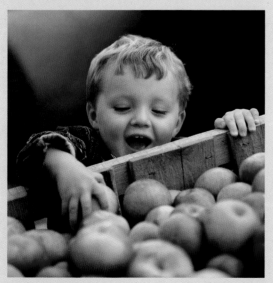

involve gorging on the latest superfood or swallowing a handful of vitamin pills, either. It's much easier and tastier than that. You just need to give some thought to what you're putting on your plate. And if you can do that, the benefits are yours for the taking. In fact, the only thing holding you back is whether you're adventurous enough to jump off the treadmill of convenience food, and, armed with your knife and fork and the information in this book, eat your way to better health. I'm well up for that and I hope you are, too.

Okay, so here's the drill – this book delivers pretty much what it says on the tin. You've got my take on the 100 foods you should be eating. Not to mention the best way to buy, prepare and cook them. Sounds easy, and by and large it is. These are foods you should be eating because they promote high-level health and because they taste good (you can relax – red wine, tea, coffee, chocolate and curry take pride of place here). Some of them you may already be an aficionado with in the kitchen. As for the flipside, there'll almost certainly be a whole lot you'll have breezed past in the supermarket without so much as a sideways glance. Everyday stuff that you might come across in the grocery section, amongst the herbs and spices, at the fish counter or, dare I say it, amidst the confectionary or even down the booze aisle. And if you don't know what hidden gems are there you'll be missing out on some top nosh.

To make life easier, I've structured the chapters to make the foods and recipes fit in with people's busy lives – not the other way around. And if your life is anything like mine and you've got to juggle a busy job, family life and still want a bit of time to hang out with your mates, this book is written for you. Happy days for anyone who lives in the real world, not the make-believe world of diet books. But above

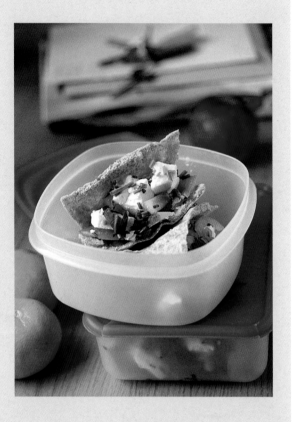

all, I hope I've made it simple. Simple enough that anyone can benefit from the information in this book. Which means there's really only one thing left to say: *Get stuck in!*

Glen.

**Glen Matten**

# Breakfast

There are quite a few of us who know that breakfast is the most important meal of the day and feast on porridge, muesli, eggs or some other equally wholesome fare, but I bet there are just as many who scoff at a healthy start or skip breakfast altogether.

Like it or not, breakfast is an important meal to get right and a chance to load-up on the right fuel to see you through the morning ahead. But a big problem is that most of us just don't have time for breakfast anymore, and if your home is anything like mine in the morning, it's full-on chaos!

Lack of time to prepare decent food is a biggie for lots of people, so I've included breakfasts for weekdays, which can be rustled up in no time or pre-prepared the night before, and weekend breakfasts for when you can take a more leisurely pace in the kitchen. But, and this is a big but, even with the quickest of these breakfasts, some of which probably take less than 5 minutes to throw together, you've still got to make a bit of time to eat it.

Saying that, I reckon when you've tasted some of these, you'll think it's well worth setting the alarm clock 15 minutes earlier...

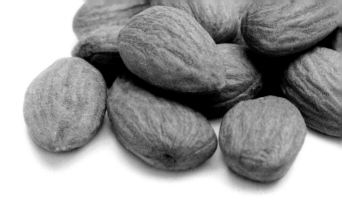

# Almonds

Nuts. All that fat. All those calories. Best avoided, right? I reckon that way of thinking is actually a bit nuts.

## Why you should be eating it

Okay, so they are calorific. And full of fat. But it's nearly all good fats. Yes, you heard right. GOOD FATS. And with almonds we're talking mostly monounsaturated fats, along with some polyunsaturated fats for good measure.

Packing all that fat you might think they'd clog your arteries quicker than you could open a packet of pralines, but check this out. The evidence actually suggests that consumption of almonds is likely to decrease the risk of heart disease, not increase it. Not only do they appear to help lower cholesterol levels, but they also contain an array of antioxidant compounds that help prevent 'bad' LDL cholesterol from becoming oxidized, making it less likely to start clogging up the inside of artery walls.

Packing their fair share of vitamins, such as vitamin E, and minerals, such as calcium and magnesium, the almond has got itself some pretty tasty credentials, shaping up as more heart-friend than heart-foe.

## How to buy it

It goes without saying that almonds are best in their natural state and not coated in a load of sugar or salt.

## How to cook it

Almonds are great for snacking, but you can use them to make fresh almond milk (which works wonders in smoothies, for making porridge, and even in place of coconut milk in curries). You can also buy a mean nut butter made from almonds, which makes a nice change from peanut butter.

## Almond milk and berry smoothie

Taking no more than a few minutes to make, this smoothie is good to go!

### Serves 2

75 g (2½ oz) blanched almonds, soaked overnight
300 ml (10½ fl oz) fresh apple juice
1 tbsp ground linseeds
1 ripe mango or 2 ripe bananas
300 g (10½ oz) berries (choose any combination of blueberries, raspberries, strawberries or blackberries – if you can't get hold of fresh ones then frozen ones are more than fine, but defrost them first)

Drain and rinse the almonds. Put them into a blender and add a little apple juice. Blend to make a smooth paste ▪ Add the remaining apple juice bit by bit and blend until you have a rich almond milk. (The key is to get rid of all the bits so it's really creamy and smooth. You're aiming for something with the consistency of its dairy counterpart) ▪ Add the linseeds, the mango or bananas and berries and blend until really smooth ▪ Serve immediately.

# Yoghurt

Yoghurt has long been the preserve of the health conscious, but is it all it's cracked up to be? Time to lift the lid and see.

## Why you should be eating it

It's no surprise that yoghurt packs loads of calcium, which is vital for bone health. Perhaps less well-known is the accumulating, albeit rather controversial, evidence that a calcium-rich diet, especially from dairy products, may have a role to play in reducing body weight and body fat. In short, a sort of anti-obesity effect, although until more research is done, it's far from a done deal.

Yoghurt also provides useful amounts of protein, which tends to be more easily digested than the protein in milk due to the fact that the bacteria used to make yoghurt do their bit by pre-digesting it. And a similar principle applies to lactose – the type of sugar found in milk – which means that individuals with an intolerance to lactose often have less problems tolerating yoghurt.

Then there's the matter of the 'friendly' bacteria that populate 'live' yoghurt. There's a whole bunch of interesting research on the potential role of specific strains of 'friendly' bacteria (or probiotics) in helping to maintain a healthy digestive system, as well as exerting a positive effect on the functioning of the immune system. But the extent to which we can expect to get these benefits from simply eating standard live yoghurt is debatable.

## How to buy it

With most people following a typical Western diet already consuming too much saturated fat, low-fat yoghurt is the obvious choice. That said, my taste buds rebel against anything too low-fat...

I go for plain natural yoghurt and give the added sugars or artificial sweeteners often found in flavoured yoghurts a wide berth, and as I don't much like the way dairy cows are treated like industrial milk-producing machines, I'm a whole lot happier with organic.

## How to cook it

Whilst you can happily use yoghurt in cooking, it's great just as it is, whether on its own, with fruit, on muesli or in smoothies.

## Banana, yoghurt and pecan smoothie

By providing a decent bit of calcium and protein from the yoghurt and 'good' fats and antioxidants from the nuts, this smoothie has a bit more going for it than a run-of-the-mill shop-bought job.

### Serves 2

4 ripe bananas
50 g (1½ oz) pecans (35 g/1 oz roughly chopped, 15 g/½ oz very finely chopped)
8 ice cubes
6 tbsp natural yoghurt
2 tbsp maple syrup
Pinch of cinnamon

Place the bananas, the roughly chopped pecan nuts, ice cubes, yoghurt and maple syrup into a blender. Blitz until you get a really smooth consistency ▪ Serve immediately in tall glasses, finishing it off by sprinkling on the remaining finely chopped pecans and a dash of cinnamon to taste.

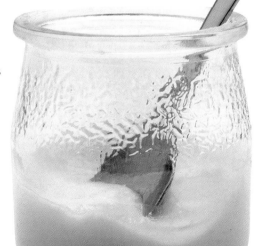

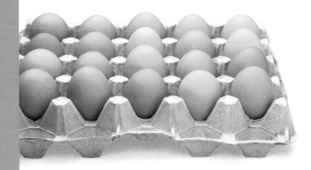

# Eggs

Eggs have had a lot of bad publicity in recent years. What with salmonella scares and all that artery choking cholesterol, their reputation has taken a right hammering. Time to set the record straight.

### Why you should be eating it

Let's start by cracking the cholesterol myth. Eggs contain lots of it, but the idea that the cholesterol we eat has a massive impact on our blood cholesterol levels is outdated. For most healthy folk, dietary cholesterol generally has a minimal effect on blood cholesterol levels. Rather it's the saturated fat in the food we eat (which eggs are relatively low in) that has a bigger impact.

All this cholesterol-phobia means we often miss out on hearing all the good stuff about eggs. Like the fact that they provide excellent quality protein. Or that those sunny yellow yolks contain the carotenoids lutein and zeaxanthin that appear to offer protection against the development of eye problems, such as age-related macular degeneration and cataracts. Or that they're one of our few dietary sources of vitamin D.

### How to buy it

When it comes to intensive factory farming of hens we all know the score, so it's free-range or organic for me every time. That's got to be worth a few pence more.

### How to cook it

Poached, boiled or scrambled are the healthiest. Happy days for those of us who like dipping toast 'soldiers' into soft boiled eggs.

## Cooked breakfast

I'm not going to pretend this is really healthy, but eating nothing but ultra healthy food would make life pretty dull. And as full cooked breakfasts go, this definitely notches up a few brownie points along the way.

Serves 2

4 good-quality butchers' sausages
A little groundnut oil
2 open capped mushrooms
A little unsalted butter
Dash of Worcestershire sauce
2 free range eggs
4 rashers lean bacon
2 tomatoes
Black pepper

### 40 mins before serving

Preheat the oven to 200°C/400°F/gas mark 6.

### 30 mins to go

Place sausages in a lightly oiled baking tray (oiled using the groundnut oil) and put in the oven.

### 15 mins to go

Spread the mushrooms with a little butter and a dash of Worcestershire sauce. Place on the baking tray alongside the sausages, giving the sausages a turn while you're there ▓ Now for the poached eggs. Place a frying pan over a gentle heat and fill with boiling water to 2.5 cm (1 in) in depth. Heat until you see a few small bubbles appearing at the bottom of the pan, then carefully break the eggs into the water, one at a time, and leave for 1 minute ▓ Turn off the heat and leave the eggs to sit for 10 minutes.

### 10 mins to go

Heat the grill to a medium heat and start grilling the bacon.

### 5 mins to go

Cut each tomato in half, season with black pepper and place under the grill with the bacon. Turn the bacon over while you're at it ▓ When the tomatoes and bacon are done, remove the eggs from the frying pan and serve it all up on warmed plates.

# Raspberries

Whilst berries get a lot of health plaudits, it always seems to be blueberries that steal the limelight. The likes of raspberries miss the party in true Cinderella style. Let's change all of that. Raspberries, you shall go to the ball!

### Why you should be eating it

Quite the vitamin C show-off, raspberries are brimming with this important antioxidant vitamin. And like many a fruit and veg, raspberries also provide generous amounts of fibre.

But to fully appreciate the health benefits of the raspberry, I reckon we need to look beyond these conventional nutrients and take a peek at the brave new world of phytochemicals. In essence, I'm talking here about the impressive array of naturally occurring compounds that are produced by plants and found in abundance in berry fruits.

These include anthocyanins, powerful antioxidants responsible for the distinctive colour of berry fruits. Whilst we only absorb small amounts of them, anthocyanins are attracting the attention of researchers interested in their potential health benefits for the ageing brain, cardiovascular health and even cancer prevention.

Of course, it doesn't end there. Berries boast numerous other phenolic compounds including proanthocyanidins, flavonols and ellagitannins, plus a whole lot more. But let's not get too carried away. Loads more research still needs to be done to better understand the role of these plant compounds in the health of us humans. In the meantime, eating a wide and diverse range of fruit and veggies looks like the smart bet.

### How to buy it

Keep your eyes peeled for fully ripe, plump, brightly coloured fruits. Generally the darker the berry the higher the levels of beneficial plant compounds are likely to be.

Rather than relying on expensive and often disappointing imports, I say make hay while the sun shines and take advantage of the raspberry season when its gets into full swing.

### How to cook it

Raspberries are great just as they are – in fruit salads, served with yoghurt, added to muesli, whizzed into a smoothie, or made into lovely home-made jam.

## Raspberry and strawberry smoothie

This simple smoothie not only tastes the business, but looks the business. First impressions and all that...

### Serves 1 (makes 300 ml/½ pint)

100 g (4 oz) fresh or defrosted raspberries
150 g (5 oz) strawberries
4 tbsp natural yoghurt
1 tbsp honey

Blitz all the ingredients together in a blender, pour into tall glasses and serve.

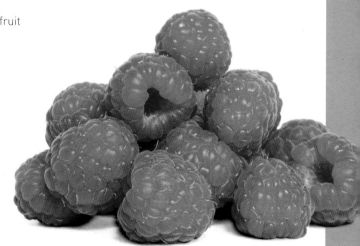

# Apples

Wise old sayings often have more than a sniff of truth about them, and we've all heard the one about an apple a day keeping the doctor away. Well there's now a decent bit of scientific evidence to support the idea that eating apples may help keep you from the doctor's door.

## Why you should be eating it

Although the data is a bit sketchy and inconsistent, apple consumption has been associated with a degree of protection against developing chronic health problems such as heart disease, some forms of cancer and asthma.

They're jam-packed with nutritional goodies such as fibre and vitamin C, but it's also likely to be the unique combination of apple phytochemicals (that's posh talk for beneficial plant compounds) that account for their health benefits.

Chief amongst these are the flavonoids, which are also found in other fruits and vegetables as well as in tea, red wine and cocoa. And whilst researchers are still trying to better understand these clever compounds, it looks likely that they may proffer some handy benefits, notably for cardiovascular health.

It's also worth remembering that many of these health-promoting compounds are found within the skin, so don't be too hasty in throwing away the peel.

## How to buy it

Whilst we have a consistent year-round supply in the supermarkets, by late summer or early autumn I'm on a mission to make the most of the locally grown, seasonal apples that abound. Bring on the knobbly bits and blemishes!

## How to cook it

There are loads of imaginative recipes using apples, but mostly they're good just as they come for snacking on, or chopped into fruit salads or muesli. And a baked apple in winter, stuffed full of dried fruits, nuts, honey and spices, is the business.

# Apple and oat muesli

This makes for a great alternative to sugar-laden breakfast cereals or those that are indistinguishable from cardboard.

### Serves 2

4 tbsp jumbo oats
1 tbsp pumpkin seeds
1 tbsp sunflower seeds
8 prunes, roughly chopped
½ glass apple juice
1 tbsp walnuts, roughly chopped
1 tbsp pecan nuts, roughly chopped
1 tbsp hazelnuts, roughly chopped
2 medium apples
1 tsp lemon juice
8 heaped tbsp natural yoghurt
½ tsp ground cinnamon
A little maple syrup (optional)

This recipe starts the night before, but it's well worth the preparation. Mix the oats, pumpkin seeds, sunflower seeds and prunes together in a bowl. Add the apple juice. Cover and refrigerate overnight (by morning the mixture should have soaked up most of the apple juice) ▪ Add the nuts and combine well ▪ Grate the apples and sprinkle with lemon juice to stop them going brown. Add to the oat mixture and combine well ▪ Spoon into individual bowls. Top with the natural yoghurt, a sprinkling of cinnamon and, if you need a hit of sweetness, a drizzle of maple syrup.

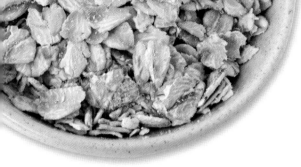

# Oats

When it comes to oats, maybe you already know your pinheads from your oatmeal. But what about your lignans from your beta-glucans?

## Why you should be eating it

It's the soluble fibre that goes by the name of beta-glucans that has sparked interest in the health benefits of oats. It soaks up cholesterol a bit like a sponge, aiding its removal from the body, accounting for the cholesterol-lowering and cardio-protective credentials of oats.

Oats are a perfect example of a wholegrain cereal, and the evidence suggests that the consumption of cereals in their unadulterated wholegrain form may promote health in numerous ways, including a reduced risk of heart disease, some cancers, diabetes and obesity.

Whilst these benefits are partly due to their fibre content, wholegrain cereals also contain a good stash of goodies such as antioxidants, phenolic compounds, plant stanols and sterols, lignans, not to mention the plain old vitamins and minerals.

Oats are also held in high esteem for their low glycemic index. This basically means they release their energy nice and slowly into the bloodstream, helping to keep energy levels stable and leaving you feeling fuller for longer.

## How to buy it

Whilst oats can come in different guises, rolled oats – the stuff of muesli and porridge fame – are widely available and cheap as chips.

## How to cook it

Oats are an archetypal breakfast cereal, never more at home than in porridge, muesli or granola. And not forgetting an indispensable ingredient in cookies, flapjacks and crumbles.

## Staffordshire oatcakes

A regional delicacy from the traditional pottery area of England, these little beauties are referred to as the Potteries' chapattis and were served from the windows of front room kitchens to ravenous workers who needed something filling, cheap and quick to eat. Sounds a bit like my house in the morning...

Makes 4 large or 8 small oatcakes

150 ml (½ pt) milk
Scant ½ tsp dried yeast
1 tsp sugar
100 g (4 oz) medium oatmeal
½ tsp salt
1 egg, beaten
Extra virgin olive oil, for frying

Warm the milk gently in a small pan until lukewarm. Pour half the warmed milk into a jug and add the yeast and sugar. Whisk and leave in a warm place until frothy ▦ Meanwhile mix the oatmeal and salt together in a bowl. Make a well in the centre and add the beaten egg. Gradually work the oatmeal into the egg, bringing it in from the sides. Stir in the milk and yeast mixture and the reserved warm milk gradually to create a smooth batter. Leave in a warm place for 30 minutes then whisk once more ▦ Heat a non-stick frying pan over a medium heat. Drop in a teaspoon of olive oil to cover the bottom of the pan. When it's smoking hot, you're ready to roll. For a large oatcake, drop in a ladle of batter so that it covers the base of the pan, or for a small one, drop in a tablespoon of batter and gently spread it out with the back of a spoon to make a pancake about 10 cm (4 in) in diameter. Wait until bubbles cover the surface of the oatcake and then turn over with a fish slice for another 30 seconds or so ▦ Serve with a topping, sweet or savoury, rolled up or left flat.

### Fillings

▦ Scrambled eggs and smoked salmon.
▦ Grated cheese and grilled sliced mushrooms, grilled to melt the cheese.
▦ Grated dark chocolate and orange zest (rolled up and lightly grilled to melt the chocolate).

# Tomatoes

We only need take a peek at the Mediterranean diet to see that tomatoes are a staple in one of the healthiest diets on the planet.

## Why you should be eating it

Tomatoes undoubtedly provide nutritious fare, packed full of vitamins, minerals and fibre, but none of those are the big reason for the avid attention they receive. That's all down to their lycopene content – the carotenoid responsible for a tomato's vibrant red colour. The lion's share of interest has focused on the potentially protective effect of this plant compound against prostate cancer.

But tomatoes aren't just man food. The evidence suggests they may also help to reduce the risk of other common cancers and cardiovascular disease, too. And just in case you were thinking of rushing out to buy lycopene in the form of a pill, eating the real thing is a much better bet. That way you'll get the whole range of nutrients and beneficial phytochemicals in the mix, such as vitamins C and E, folate, other carotenoids and polyphenols, and that's just for starters.

If you want to maximize the amount of lycopene you get from your tomatoes, it's well worth knowing that our bodies absorb loads more from cooked and processed tomatoes than from raw ones. And consuming a little bit of oil or fat at the same time also helps.

## How to buy it

Look out for tomatoes that are a bright, deep red colour. That way you'll be bagging those with a higher lycopene content.

## How to cook it

Tomatoes make for an indispensable salad ingredient, and when it comes to cooking, there's not much you can't do with tomatoes, be it fresh or tinned. Think soups, stews and pasta sauces. And remember that olive oil, herbs, onions and garlic make for great companions.

## Roasted cherry tomatoes on pesto toast

The key to making this look as funky as possible is to cook and serve the cherry tomatoes on the vine.

Per person

8–10 cherry tomatoes on the vine
1 tbsp extra virgin olive oil
Sea salt and black pepper
2 thick slices wholemeal (whole-wheat)
    or granary bread
2 tbsp fresh pesto (see page 71)

Evenly coat the tomatoes with the olive oil and a little sea salt and black pepper ▤ Roast on a baking tray for 10 minutes at 200°C/400°F/gas mark 6 until the skins begin to shrivel ▤ Meanwhile, toast the bread on both sides and spread one side with the pesto ▤ Carefully place half of the tomatoes on to each slice of toast and season with lots of black pepper.

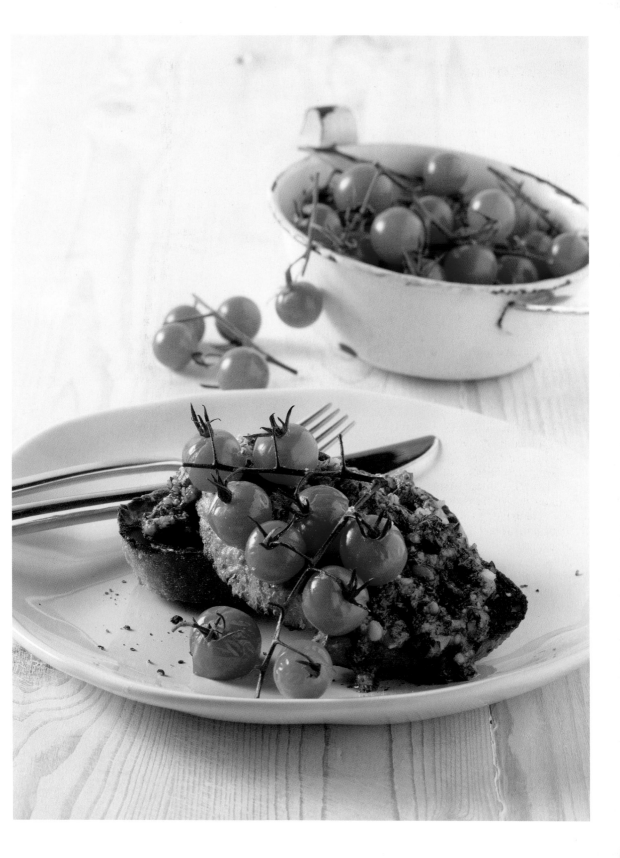

# The munchies

I do my best to eat three decent meals a day and I usually just about manage it. But most days don't run like clockwork and my guess is that the same is true for most people. That's why I really like the idea of grazing. Regular pit-stops to top-up on nutritious fare has got to be a whole lot better for us than skipping meals and following erratic eating patterns. Don't get me wrong, if you've got time to prepare and eat three square meals a day, good for you. Make the most of it. But if I've got a hectic day ahead of me and still want to make it to footie with my mates after work, then grazing definitely works for me.

Having said that, as with many a great principle, things can go decidedly pear-shaped in practice. And that's because proper, healthy snacks for grazing aren't particularly easy to come by when you're out and about doing your thing. 'Snack food' is pretty much synonymous with high sugar (think confectionary) or high salt (think crisps). And that completely defeats the object.

So that really only leaves one option and that's to DIY your snacks. At its simplest, this might mean slinging a couple of pieces of fruit and a bag of nuts into your bag on your way out the door (and just about everyone can manage that). But if you're up for a bit more of a culinary adventure, you could face the day packing some of the tasty morsels I've lined up for you in this chapter.

What more can I say. Happy grazing!

# Bananas

There are no great shakes when it comes to bananas. Just a good solid all-rounder. And that's what I like about them.

## Why you should be eating it

Bananas offer up some useful nutrients, notably vitamins C and B6, and the bit of general knowledge trivia that just about everyone knows – potassium.

I'd be surprised if there are many folk out there who aren't aware that too much sodium (salt) can cause problems with high blood pressure, a big risk for stroke. But probably less well known is that potassium has the opposite effect and can actually help lower pressure. And eating fruit regularly, including bananas, is just about one of the best ways to bump up potassium intake.

Bananas also provide a good bit of fibre, including a less well known type called fructo-oligosaccharide (we'll stick with FOS for short). Whilst FOS is largely indigestible to us humans, it provides a veritable feast for the 'friendly' bacteria that inhabit our digestive system. That makes it a 'prebiotic', which basically means food for our good bugs. Happy days for digestive health.

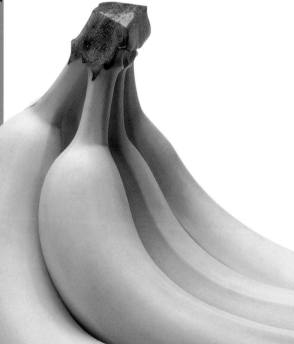

## How to buy it

It all depends how you like your 'nanas. I reckon they're best when they've ripened to the point where they're still yellow but with the first signs of a few tiny brown flecks. But hey, each to their own.

## How to cook it

With no cooking required, and individually wrapped by Mother Nature herself, they make for perfect grazing fare.

# Banana and walnut muffin

Okay, I'll be honest with you. This muffin isn't totally healthy. There's a bit of butter and sugar in the mix. But at the end of the day, there's only so much you can do to a muffin before it stops being a muffin and turns into something so 'healthy' that no one wants to eat it anymore. Compare the ingredients here to what you'll be getting in a pre-made shop-bought job, and I reckon we've got a pretty good thing going on.

### For 8 muffins

150 g (5 oz) rice flour
1 tsp baking powder
½ tsp cinnamon powder
½ tsp nutmeg, grated
40 g (1½ oz) molasses sugar
1 large egg
1 tsp vanilla extract
125 g (4½ oz) natural yoghurt
50 g (2 oz) butter, melted and cooled
2 large, ripe bananas, mashed
50 g (2 oz) walnuts, chopped

Pre-heat the oven to 190°C/ 375°F/gas mark 5 ■ Sift the flour, baking powder, cinnamon and nutmeg into a large mixing bowl and mix in the molasses ■ In another bowl, whisk together the egg, vanilla extract, yoghurt and melted butter ■ Combine the wet and dry ingredients and mix in the mashed banana and walnuts ■ Spoon the mixture into non-stick muffin tins and bake for 20-25 minutes.

# Celery

Celery is synonymous with slimming due to its miniscule calorie content. But there is more to food than calorie counting, and celery goes large in other ways.

## Why you should be eating it

Whilst not exactly over-flowing with nutrients, celery serves up a decent bit of the blood pressure-lowering mineral potassium.

I'm sure you don't need me to tell you that eating a variety of fruit and veg confers numerous health advantages, but one of the unsung benefits is the effect they have on helping us stay trim. Veggies such as celery are packed full of fibre and, with a high water content, tend to leave us feeling full despite being inherently low in calories. Substituting calorie-laden high fat or high sugar foods with fresh veggies is an entirely healthy way of reducing energy intake.

No self-respecting vegetable would be without its fair share of beneficial phytochemicals. In the case of celery, it contains two different types of flavones called apigenin and luteolin, which researchers are investigating for their potential anti-inflammatory, anti-oxidant and anti-cancer properties, although loads more research is still to be done to unravel their precise health benefits.

## How to buy it

Celery is available pretty much all year round, but be on the look-out for local produce when it's available. Buy celery that is really crisp, firm and fresh. If it's looking all floppy and bendy, steer clear.

## How to cook it

Celery can add some serious crunch to salads. It also works well in soups, casseroles and stews, where you can happily use the tougher outer stalks. And don't just sling out the leaves, which can be used just like you would herbs in salads.

## Celery bites

This might take longer than opening a bag of crisps, but not a whole lot longer.

All you need for this are some celery stalks and a topping.

To prepare the celery stalks, wash, slice off the bottom and top and cut into 5 cm (2 in) pieces. Then you just spoon or spread on your topping. Here's my favourite.

## Roasted cumin topping

For 1 celery stalk (3-4 bites)

1 tsp cumin seeds
2 tbsp low fat cream cheese
Lemon juice to taste

Heat a small pan and dry roast the cumin seeds for a couple of minutes, tossing them occasionally, until they are slightly brown. Take care not to burn them. Remove from the heat and grind to a coarse powder in a coffee grinder or pestle and mortar ▧ Mix the cumin with the cream cheese and lemon juice, to taste, and spoon into the prepared celery pieces.

# Red grapes

Whilst I'll happily tuck into white grapes, it's the compounds within the skins of red grapes that are the real attention grabbers.

## Why you should be eating it

Red grapes offer up a plentiful source of antioxidants and are brimming with vitamin C. But the real interest is in the heaps of phytochemicals found in red grapes in the form of polyphenolic compounds. And it's these clever plant compounds, largely derived from the skin of red grapes, which accounts for a lot of the fuss about the health benefits of red wine.

Notable amongst these are plentiful amounts of flavonoids, including the likes of anthocyanins and proanthocyanidins. And whilst we don't absorb them very efficiently, including plenty of flavonoid-rich foods in the diet appears to bestow health benefits such as a reduced risk of heart disease. Researchers are also interested in other possible positive effects such as retarding the decline in brain function as we age, although there's still plenty more to be uncovered on this.

Another polyphenolic compound found in red grapes includes the much-hyped resveratrol, widely touted for its cardio-protective properties and other health enhancing attributes such as inhibiting cancer development and promoting longevity. But before we get swept away with all of this, it must be said that most of the research at present comes from experiments in test tubes or animals and not real life humans, so should be taken with a good pinch of salt until more is known.

## How to buy it

Obviously, we want fresh looking specimens. And the darker the colour the higher the levels of beneficial phytochemicals are likely to be.

An alternative way to take on board good levels of these beneficial compounds is through purple grape juice, in effect a bit like a booze-free version of red wine.

## How to cook it

Red grapes are perfect for snacking, just as they come, or as a welcome addition to fruit salads.

# Ridiculously easy fruit salad

Fruit makes for a great in-between meal snack, and here's a good way to make it a tad more interesting. The whole point of this fruit salad is that once you've prepared it you can store it in the fridge and dip in and out of it as you please. If you want to liven things up, I've included a humdinger of a dip, too.

Serves 2

FOR THE FRUIT SALAD
½ a small cantaloupe melon, halved, with seeds and skin removed
50 g (1¾ oz) blueberries
50 g (1¾ oz) red and green seedless grapes
50 g (1¾ oz) strawberries, halved

FOR THE MANGO DIP
1 ripe mango
4 tbsp natural Greek yoghurt
1 tbsp maple syrup

To make the fruit salad, cut the melon into bite-sized chunks and then carefully mix all of the ingredients together ■ To make the dip, peel the mango and cut the flesh into chunks. Add to a blender along with the Greek yoghurt and maple syrup. Blend until smooth ■ Eat straight away, or store in a plastic tub in the fridge to have on hand for between-meal munchies.

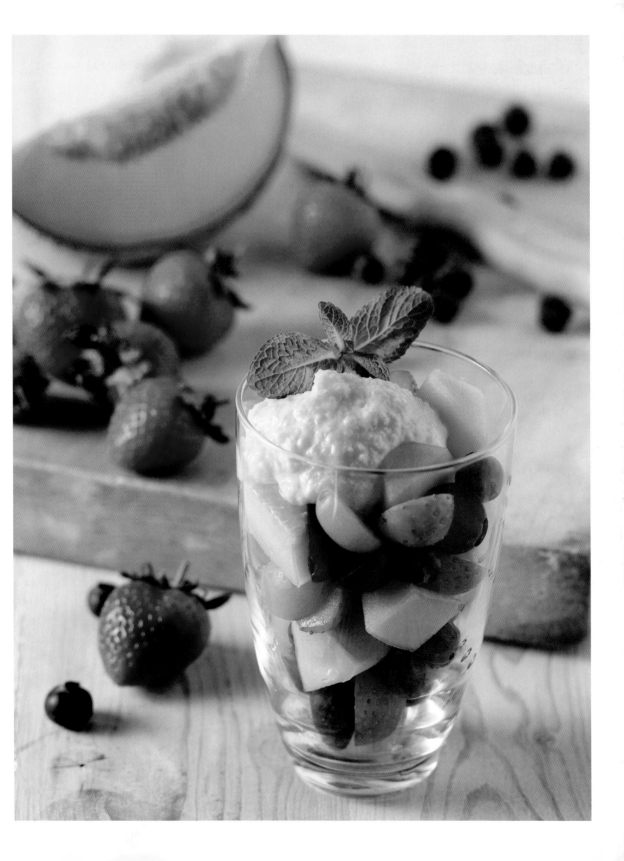

# Cashew nuts

The low-fat mantra has been drummed into most of us, in which case you'd have thought that nuts, bulging with fat, should by rights be struck off the menu. Well, read on...

## Why you should be eating it

Whilst cashews do tend to have a lower fat content than most other nuts, they're still a high fat food. But here's the deal-breaker. Most of it comes in the form of unsaturated fats ('good' fats). And these are altogether different to the saturated fats that predominate in other high fat foods such as processed snacks and junk food.

When it comes to heart health, nuts have a pretty impressive track record, associated with lowering cholesterol levels and reducing the risk of heart disease. Indeed, a review of the evidence from some major epidemiological studies showed that the risk of coronary heart disease was 37 per cent lower for those consuming nuts more than four times per week, compared to those who didn't consume nuts at all.

Whilst the favourable balance of fats in nuts is undoubtedly an important factor, there's lots more going on behind the scenes. Nuts are high in antioxidants, fibre, vitamins, minerals and phytosterols, the latter being naturally occurring compounds that interfere with the absorption of cholesterol in the gut, and so helping to lower cholesterol levels in the bloodstream.

BUT, won't they make you fat? The evidence shows that this doesn't appear to happen. If anything, people who regularly consume nuts are slimmer than those who don't. Nuts have a strong satiety effect, basically making you feel full and suppressing hunger. If that means they end up replacing less healthy energy-dense foods, which are high in sugar or bad fats, then that's a total bonus.

## How to buy it

Plain and natural. Not encased in sugar.

## How to cook it

Cashews make for great snacks. You could also try tossing them into stir-fries and salads. And if you want an alternative to peanut butter, give cashew nut butter a whirl.

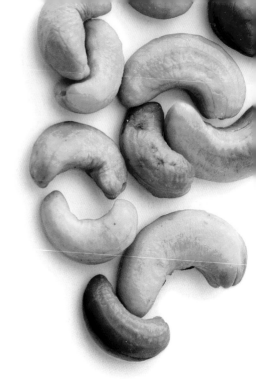

## Honey-roasted cashew nuts

There is one problem with this recipe. Once they're made, I can't stop eating them.

100 g (3½ oz) cashew nuts, roughly broken
Zest of an unwaxed orange
2 tsp ground mixed spice
¼ tsp ground cinnamon
2 tsp clear honey

Put the cashew nuts, orange zest, mixed spice, cinnamon and honey into a bowl and mix well, making sure the cashews are evenly coated ■ Transfer to a baking tray and bake in a preheated oven at 200°C/400°F/gas mark 6 for 8–10 minutes. Give them an occasional stir to make sure they don't burn ■ Transfer to a dish to cool and go crunchy.

# Pumpkin seeds

Start nibbling on a handful of these at work and I bet it's less than 10 seconds before your workmates will start muttering something about rabbit food. Definitely not man food, that's for sure. Or is it...?

### Why you should be eating it

Much like other nuts and seeds, pumpkin seeds are a good source of minerals such as magnesium, manganese, iron, zinc and copper. But they are a right fatty of a food with somewhere in the region of two thirds of their calories coming from fat. No reason for panic though. The lion's share of these fats come in the form of the healthy unsaturated type.

Pumpkin seeds are also a rich source of phytosterols. These clever compounds, which are prevalent in nuts, seeds and unrefined plant oils, are infamous for their ability to reduce cholesterol levels, thereby helping to lower the risk of heart disease. Other suggested benefits include decreasing the risk of certain types of cancer and enhancing the immune system.

Munching on a few pumpkin seeds certainly doesn't win any awards for macho behaviour. It's hardly like ripping in to a juicy slab of bloody steak. But pumpkin seeds may just turn out to be man food after all, with a folk tradition (although scant scientific evidence, it must be said) suggesting that they could help alleviate some of the symptoms of benign prostatic hyperplasia, or BPH for short – a non-cancerous enlargement of the prostate gland that's pretty common in older men.

### How to buy it

As with other nuts and seeds, I'd be looking to pick up pumpkin seeds from a shop with a pretty decent turnover of stock to ensure freshness. And to protect all those unsaturated fats from going rancid, it would be ideal to keep them stored in an airtight container in the fridge.

### How to cook it

Pumpkin seeds can be sprinkled on muesli or porridge just as they are, or better still ground up with other seeds such as sunflower seeds, sesame seeds and linseeds. They're also a good addition to a leafy salad for a bit of crunch, especially if lightly toasted first.

## Toasted tamari seeds

Are you ready for this? Rabbit food it isn't! As well as a neat snack to have handy when you're on the go, these tasty little morsels make for an ideal something to nibble on when friends come round for food or drinks. They're also the business sprinkled on to salads, soups, even steamed or stir-fried veggies.

2 handfuls of sunflower seeds
2 handfuls of pumpkin seeds
2 tbsp tamari soy sauce
1 tsp garam masala (optional)
Pinch of cayenne pepper (optional)

Mix the seeds with the tamari before toasting under a hot grill. (For a bit of pizzazz, you could add a teaspoon of garam masala powder.) Stir regularly to prevent them from burning – about 4 minutes should do it ■ Allow to cool. To add some fire, sprinkle the seeds with a dusting of cayenne pepper.

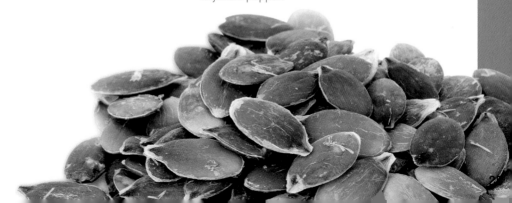

# Oatcakes

Oatcakes have a reputation for being a bit 'holier than thou', but they're cheap as chips, nutritious and perfectly designed for snacking.

## Why you should be eating it

Being made from oatmeal, they boast an impressively low GI (glycemic index). For those not in the know, this means that they're a slow-releasing energy food. They're perfect for keeping energy levels on an even keel, as well as promoting a satisfying feeling of fullness that discourages between-meal attacks of the munchies.

Eating more in the way of fibre-rich, low GI wholegrains, as opposed to faster-releasing refined 'white' versions, may carry with it the additional longer term health benefits of a reduced risk of heart disease, diabetes and obesity.

To further big-up their healthy-heart credentials they also contain a type of soluble fibre by the name of beta-glucan, renowned for its cholesterol-lowering properties. It does this by binding to cholesterol and helping to eliminate it from the body.

## How to buy it

Oatcakes are a straightforward, basic, rustic food. So whichever brand you go for, they should have a high percentage of oatmeal and not a long list of other ingredients.

## How to cook it

On their own, oatcakes notch up close to zero on the taste-o-meter. But combine them with a luscious topping and we're talking business.

## Ten ways with oatcakes

The mission: To turn an oatcake into a lip-smacker of a snack. Try any of these and it'll definitely be mission accomplished.

- Spread a thin layer of tahini on to your oatcakes and top with a few slices of roast (bell) peppers, either your own creation or the sort that come from a jar – either will work well.

- Slather on a decent helping of liver pâté and add a sliced cornichon or gherkin (pickle).

- Spoon over a layer of pesto (see page 71 for a home-made version) and top with avocado and tomato slices.

- Oatcakes and hummus were made for each other. Give the Spice-topped Hummus on page 111 a go and see if you agree.

- Packed with nutrient-rich avocados, guacamole is a real winner in the healthy food stakes. But steer well clear of the tasteless shop-bought stuff and have a go at making your own (see page 108) to reap the maximum health rewards.

- My Butterbean and Miso Pâté (see page 35) will have even the hardiest of meat eaters converted to this simple veggie fare.

- While not low fat, cheese does pack a punch when in comes to calcium and a little bit of what we fancy does us good, right? So try some soft goat's cheese with a scattering of chives or spring onions (scallions) for a decadent topping that would be great for pre-dinner nibbles.

- We all know that fish is good for us, so why not combine the health benefits of wholegrains with omega 3-rich oily fish and spread on a bit of mackerel pâté for a nutrient-packed snack.

- Peanut butter and mashed banana is a perfect combination, or you could give any other nut butter a go.

- To satisfy a sweet craving without loading up on refined sugars, add a dollop of Greek yoghurt, top with a few raspberries and drizzle over a bit of honey.

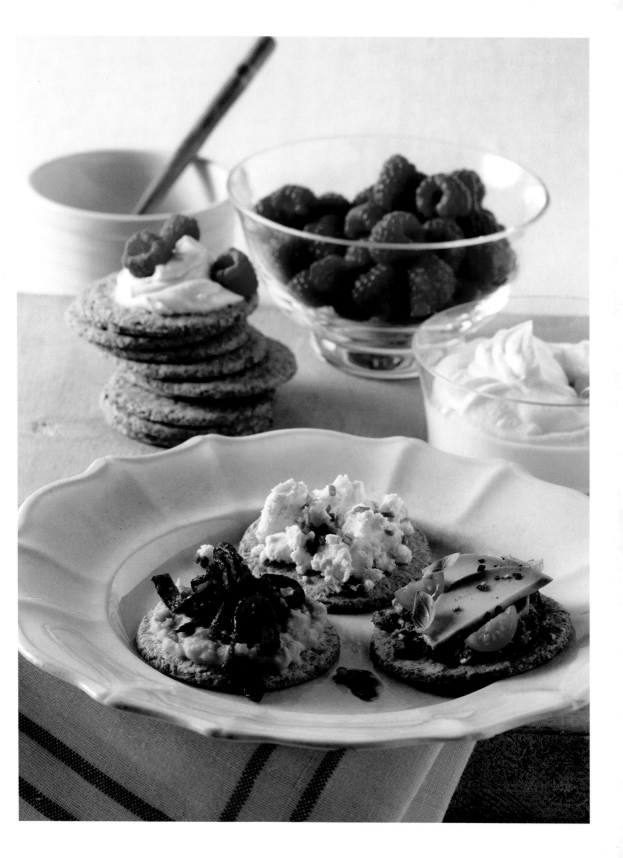

# 3

# Lunch on the go

When push comes to shove, it's a whole lot harder to make healthy choices when you're out and about compared with being at home. The big problem is that most of us spend a hefty chunk of time at work, and when it comes to getting some half-decent grub at lunchtime, genuinely healthy choices are a bit thin on the ground. Sure, some staff canteens offer pretty decent fare and there are some great salad bars, delis and sandwich shops around – if you know where to find them. But by and large, I reckon for a lot of people it's a case of eating the same drab cheese or tuna sandwich and bag of crisps, whilst stuck at their desk, hunched over their PC, trying not to get too many crumbs in between the keys.

Truth is, we could be eating a whole lot better at work. I've even devised a foolproof (and in no way whatsoever) scientific formula to solve the problem:

A bit of imagination + 15 minutes prep time + a trusty lunchbox = a mighty fine packed lunch

So dust down your lunchbox and get ready to roll. My guess is you won't look back.

# Watercress

It's about time watercress had a well-earned promotion from the lowly position of decorative garnish.

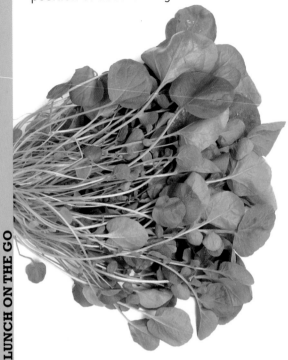

## Why you should be eating it

Watercress is actually a member of the cruciferous family of vegetables, which means it contains significant amounts of a group of phytochemicals called glucosinolates (notably gluconasturtin). These plant compounds are broken down to isothiocyanates when we eat them, and they're thought to be one of the main reasons why diets high in cruciferous vegetables are associated with a reduced risk of several cancers. In the case of watercress, it's the unique mustard oil with the snappy name phenethyl isothiocyanate (or PEITC for short) that's attracted the most attention to date.

Watercress is also bursting at the seams with carotenoids, notably lutein and zeaxanthin. Present in the retina and lens of the eye, these two plant compounds are likely candidates for protection against age-related macular degeneration and cataracts.

Watercress also contains more than its fair share of the traditional vitamins and minerals. In particular, a noteworthy cocktail of nutrients important for building and maintaining strong bones, including calcium, vitamin K and vitamin C.

## How to buy it

Watercress can be found in bags or bunches in just about any supermarket. Given the choice, I'd go for the seasonal, organic stuff if I can get my hands on it.

## How to cook it

We don't have to complicate everything by cooking it. Watercress makes for great salads, offering a bit of variety to lettuce, and is definitely something different to shove in your sarnie or a pitta bread. Of course you can cook watercress too and it makes a wicked soup.

## Watercress, orange and pumpkin seed salad

Here's a great alternative to expensive pre-packaged salads, and it can be knocked-up in less time than it takes to queue at the supermarket – bonus!

Serves 4

4 oranges
2 bags or large bunches watercress, washed
4 tbsp toasted pumpkin seeds

FOR THE DRESSING
2 tbsp extra virgin olive oil
2 tsp runny honey
Juice of 1 lemon

Slice the top and bottom off of each orange so that they stand steady on the chopping board. Take a small knife and cut away the peel and pith so that you're just left with the orange flesh. Cut out each individual segment with a knife ■ Roughly chop the watercress and gently combine with the orange segments in a bowl. Mix together the dressing and drizzle over the salad ■ Sprinkle over the pumpkin seeds and serve.

# Coriander (Cilantro)

I'm up for using herbs a bit more frequently in cooking. Not only to big things up in the taste department, but also to add some useful nutrients in to the mix.

### Why you should be eating it

Okay, so we're never going to eat herbs in the same quantity as we would a vegetable, nor would we want to. But seeing that most of our diets are pretty low on fruit and veg anyway, I reckon anything that adds a bit of greenery along the way is well worth giving a whirl.

And fresh coriander does actually share many of the nutritional properties we would typically associate with green leafy veg. For example, it contains good levels of antioxidants such as beta carotene and vitamin C. Indeed, when scientists have measured the antioxidant value of lots of different foods using something called the oxygen radical absorbance capacity, or ORAC for short, fresh coriander leaf measured up pretty well against other antioxidant rich fruits and veg. Just like green leafy veg, fresh coriander also provides useful amounts of bone-building vitamin K and homocysteine-lowering folate.

So all-in-all, with a lack of the green leafy stuff in our diets, I reckon a generous sprinkling of coriander here and there goes at least some way to making up for it.

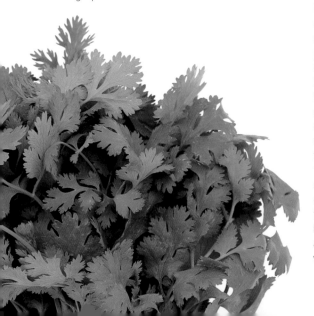

### How to buy it

Look for fresh, lush green leaves that show no signs of wilting.

### How to cook it

Coriander is at its best in salsas, curries and soups, and can even be used to add a bit of interest to salads. For a bigger hit, you can blitz it up to make a fresh coriander pesto (see page 106). For maximum flavour always add it towards the end of cooking.

## Carrot, coriander and ginger soup

With a bit of forward planning you can get away from the monotony of cheese sandwiches. Come on, try something different!

Serves 4

1 tbsp coriander seeds
1 tbsp extra virgin olive oil
1 large onion, finely chopped
1 large garlic clove, crushed
900 g (2 lb) carrots, scrubbed and chopped
5 cm (2 in) piece of fresh ginger, peeled and grated
1 litre (2 pt) vegetable stock
100 g (4 oz) red lentils, washed and drained
Black pepper
4 tbsp fresh coriander (cilantro), chopped

Heat a small pan over a high heat and dry roast the coriander seeds just until they start to pop. Remove and grind to a coarse powder in a coffee grinder or pestle and mortar ■ Heat the oil in the same pan over a medium heat and add the onion and garlic. Fry for a few minutes until the onion becomes translucent and soft ■ Add the ground coriander seeds, stir well and fry for a further minute ■ Add the carrots and grated ginger and mix well. Cover and cook over a moderate heat so it gently sizzles until the carrots begin to soften (this should take about 15 minutes), stirring halfway through ■ Add the stock and lentils and simmer for 20 minutes until the carrots are tender and lentils are soft ■ Leave to cool for a couple of minutes and then blend until smooth ■ Add the fresh coriander and serve. Or leave to cool and refrigerate. It's then ready to re-heat and take to work in a flask the next day.

# Quinoa

Quinoa has been the preserve of hardcore healthfood enthusiasts for many years, and while probably not a regular feature on the menu in most households, it's well worth giving it a go.

## Why you should be eating it

Quinoa provides decent amounts of protein and a good spread of minerals such as iron and magnesium. Pound for pound, it punches above its weight compared with the nutrients found in most other grains.

What marks quinoa out from the bunch is that its relatively high protein is made up of a desirable balance of amino acids (the building blocks of protein). This makes it much more 'complete' as a protein food compared with other grains, hence its popularity amongst vegetarians. It's also gluten-free, making it suitable for individuals with Coeliac disease or gluten intolerance.

## How to buy it

For a long time, quinoa could only be tracked down in the most wholesome of healthfood stores, but it's now widely available in most supermarkets.

It comes not only in its 'wholegrain' form, but also as flakes and flour, so there's no shortage of options (although I'm still not convinced quinoa flake porridge can ever taste good...).

## How to cook it

Quinoa needs a really thorough rinse under cold running water before cooking. A fine-meshed sieve should do just fine. Then you're ready to roll. You can cook quinoa like you would brown rice, and the best way of doing that is to use one part quinoa to two parts water. Bring this to the boil, then cover and simmer until all the water has gone, roughly 12–15 minutes.

# Lynn's citrus quinoa

I've got to be honest, I'd never much enjoyed quinoa. That is, until I tasted this. Lynn is one of the amazing volunteers who helps out with the diet and behaviour projects I run with local kids. And in coming up with this little number, she proved that quinoa can taste the business. Pack this away in a plastic tub and it makes for a great at-the-desk breakfast.

Serves 4

225 g (8 oz) quinoa
3 star anise
3 unwaxed oranges
1 unwaxed lemon
½ unwaxed lime
175 g (6 oz) dried apricots, chopped
100 g (3½ oz) sultanas (golden raisins)
1 tsp ground cinnamon
3 tbsp runny honey

Cook the quinoa in a pan of boiling water with the star anise for 12–15 minutes (until cooked but still slightly chewy). Strain and leave to cool. Remove the star anise and set aside for decoration ▧ Finely grate the rind of 2 oranges, the lemon and half a lime. Mix in a bowl with the dried apricots and sultanas ▧ Squeeze the juice from 1 orange, half a lemon and half a lime and add to the dried fruit mixture ▧ Add the cinnamon and honey and mix well ▧ Place the cooled quinoa into a bowl and add the dried fruit and citrus mixture, stirring gently ▧ Make orange slices by cutting the top and bottom from both oranges and resting them bottom down on a chopping board. Following the contours of the orange, slice off the skin and remove the pith. Cut out each individual segment with a knife. Gently stir the orange slices into the quinoa mixture ▧ Lovely served with a big splodge of Greek yoghurt and a star anise for decoration.

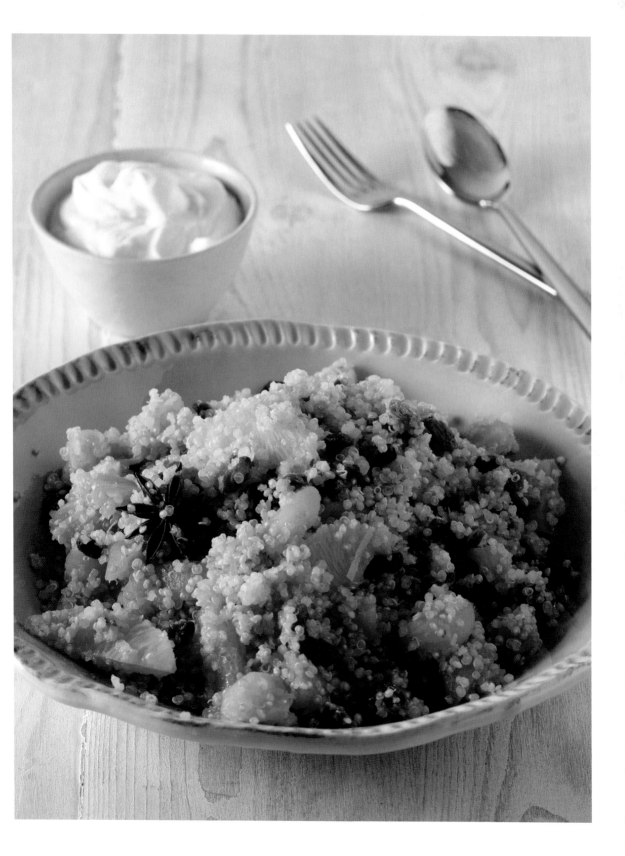

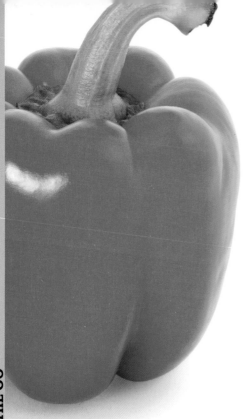

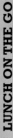

And they're also blessed with decent amounts of B-vitamins, notably folate and B6, which work together to help control blood levels of homocysteine, a substance we all produce but in high amounts is implicated in increasing the risk of heart disease.

## How to buy it

Be on the lookout for firm, shiny, deeply coloured, wrinkle-free peppers. Whilst all colours of peppers are to be encouraged, it's of interest that red peppers contain significantly more carotenoids and vitamin C than their green counterparts. But hey, at the end of the day, they're all good.

## How to cook it

Peppers are great raw in salads or as vegetable crudités, with the sweeter yellow, orange and red peppers working best. And there's no end to their use in cooking: stuffed, roasted, pizza toppings, vegetable kebabs, stir-fries, casseroles... you get the picture.

## Feta, sun-dried tomato and herb packed pitta

Time to give the bog-standard cheese sandwich a well deserved make-over.

### Serves 1

2 wholemeal (whole-wheat) pitta breads
75 g (3 oz) feta cheese, cubed
½ red (bell) pepper, finely sliced
¼ red onion, finely sliced
20 g (¾ oz) sun-dried tomatoes, rehydrated and finely sliced
20 g (¾ oz) rocket (arugula)
10 black olives, pitted and halved
10 basil leaves, shredded
½ avocado, cut into bite sized cubes
1 tbs extra virgin olive oil
Black pepper

Gently toast the pitta breads ■ Combine all the other ingredients together in a mixing bowl, drizzle with the olive oil and season with black pepper ■ Carefully pack the mixture into the pittas and serve.

# Peppers (Bell peppers)

Let me tell you something I don't like: the heavily promoted idea that if we just eat a certain 'superfood' it will solve all our health problems and keep us forever young. And something I do like: the idea that we should eat a rainbow of different brightly coloured fruits and veggies every day. Coming in yellow, orange, green and red, bell peppers fit the bill.

## Why you should be eating it

We tend to associate vitamin C with fruit such as oranges or kiwi fruits, but bell peppers are a stunner in the vitamin C stakes. Just half of a small red pepper will comfortably match, and probably exceed, an adult's recommended daily requirement for this important antioxidant vitamin. That bell peppers (mainly the red ones) also contain top notch levels of carotenoids, notably beta carotene, gives a further boost to their antioxidant credentials.

# Butter (Lima) beans

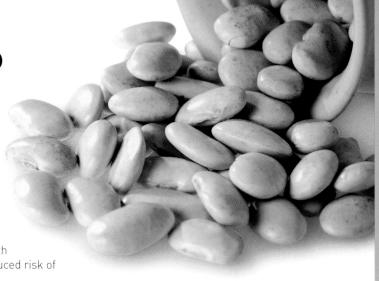

I reckon it's time to come clean and spill the beans on.....err.....beans.

## Why you should be eating it

Butter beans are packed full of protein, complex carbohydrates and fibre. And that makes for a pretty healthy combo, with frequent consumption of beans associated with reduced cholesterol levels and a reduced risk of heart disease and diabetes.

Butter beans boast an impressively low Glycaemic Index (GI). In effect, this means that they provide a slow and gradual release of energy into the bloodstream, conducive to stable energy levels. Diets based on low GI foods may also help to prevent or better manage diabetes, whilst potentially reducing the risk of heart disease. It also tends to mean they'll be more satiating, helping us feel fuller for longer and lessening the chance of an attack of the between-meal munchies.

Beans are also a good source of resistant starch. This is a type of starch that remains undigested until it comes into contact with the friendly bugs in our large intestine, which have a field day fermenting it to produce some useful substances such as short-chain fatty acids, which promote the health of the colon.

And let's not forget that as well as containing good amounts of the traditional vitamins and minerals, beans also contain a whole shooting match of other bioactive components, such as cholesterol-lowering phytosterols, oligosaccharides, isoflavones and phytic acid, which we're only just beginning to understand the potential health benefits of.

## How to buy it

If time is tight and convenience is important, you can cut out the middleman and buy them pre-cooked in a can, avoiding those with added sugar or salt. Of course, you can always buy them in their dried form, which require lengthy pre-soaking and cooking.

## How to cook it

Butter beans make for a hearty addition to soups and casseroles, and are great mashed up into a chunky and funky pâté.

## Butter bean and miso pâté

Whilst I'm a big fan of a really meaty pâté, I'm equally happy to tuck into a veggie version. Providing it comes big on flavour that is. And this one fits the bill perfectly.

### Serves 2

1 x 410 g (14½ oz) can butter (lima) beans, drained and rinsed
2 tbsp extra virgin olive oil
1 tbsp miso paste
½ an unwaxed lime, juice and zest
4 medium spring onions (scallions), trimmed and finely chopped
1 garlic clove, crushed
¼ tsp dried chilli flakes
Black pepper

Stick all the ingredients into a mixing bowl ■ Get to work on it with a potato masher, giving it the occasional mix around to ensure the ingredients are evenly distributed ■ It won't take long before you've got a pâté with a fairly course texture, like a courser version of mashed potato ■ Serve the pâté on fresh bread, toast, wholegrain crackers, oat cakes, as a jacket potato filling, or as a dip with vegetable crudités.

# Butternut squash

When it comes to starchy veg it can sometimes seem like there's no world beyond the potato. Don't get me wrong, I love a good spud, but I'm also up for a bit more variety in our diets.

### Why you should be eating it

Butternut squash is a decent antioxidant all-rounder, containing a good hit of carotenoids, along with a respectable bit of vitamin C for good measure.

Butternut squash stashes loads of beta carotene, which accounts for the distinctive orange-colouring of its flesh. Not only can the body use beta carotene as a precursor to make vitamin A, it also acts as an antioxidant. And observational studies have consistently shown that a high dietary intake of beta-carotene is associated with a reduced risk of serious health problems such as heart disease and cancer.

However, don't be fooled into thinking you can skip the food bit and take a beta carotene pill instead. The evidence shows us that won't work and may even do more harm than good, especially if you smoke. But getting your beta carotene from fruits and veggies means you also take on board a complex and diverse range of other beneficial plant compounds. Isolating just one of those and taking them as a high dose pill is most definitely not the way to do it.

### How to buy it

I'd give it a quick once over to check that it's firm and fresh and not showing signs of age such as squidgy bits of decay or mould.

### How to cook it

When it comes to butternut squash, I've got three words to say: bake, roast, soup.

## Butternut squash soup

Unveil a flask full of this winter warmer at work and watch your workmates drool.

Serves 4

1 tbsp olive oil
1 tsp mustard seeds
1 tsp cumin seeds
1 large onion, diced
1 garlic clove, crushed
1 celery stick, chopped
1 red chilli, deseeded and chopped
1 butternut squash (roughly 1 kg/2¼ lbs), peeled, deseeded and cut into chunks
850 ml (1½ pts) water
200 g (7 oz) creamed coconut, roughly chopped
Sea salt and black pepper

Heat the oil in a large pan. Throw in the mustard and cumin seeds and stir until they begin to pop ■ Add the onion, garlic, celery and chilli and cook for a further 2 minutes ■ Add the squash, water and creamed coconut, bring to the boil and simmer, stirring occasionally, until the squash is really soft and tender ■ Transfer to a blender and process until smooth ■ Season to taste and serve. Or cool and refrigerate, ready to re-heat and take to work in a flask the next day.

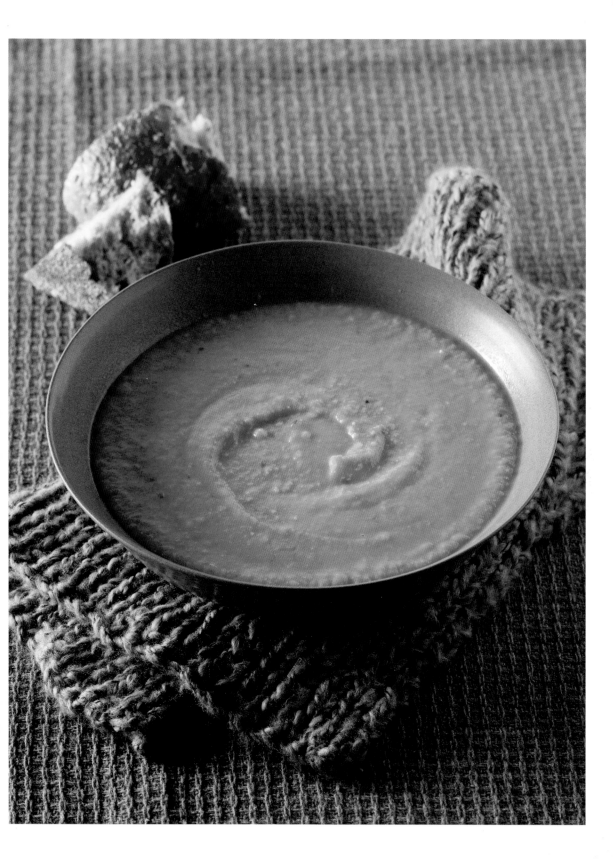

# Rye bread

I admit that rye bread has got a reputation for inducing jaw ache, and that some loaves are so heavy and dense that you're at risk of putting your back out when you lift them off the shelf. But there are plenty of wholegrain rye loaves that taste more than decent, too, so don't be too quick to write them off.

## Why you should be eating it

Wholegrain rye bread is a perfect way to reap the health benefits associated with consumption of wholegrain cereals. This not insignificant list includes a reduced risk of heart disease, certain cancers, diabetes, and to put a big, fat, juicy, cherry on top, obesity. Whilst it's never easy to prove these things for sure, it offers a strong case for ditching the refined 'white' versions.

Wholegrain rye bread contributes generous amounts of dietary fibre, something most folk eating modern diets simply don't get enough of. Obvious benefits of a higher intake of fibre include improved digestive health and reduced risk of colon cancer, along with the added bonus of heart disease protection.

But wholegrains have a whole lot more good stuff going on, containing hundreds of beneficial plant compounds, antioxidants, resistant starch and oligosaccharides, phytoestrogens such as lignans, and plant sterols. And that's before we even think about the more conventional nutrients such as the numerous essential minerals and B-vitamins. And, a bit like fruits and vegetables, it's this complex matrix of nutrients that ultimately accounts for rye's health promoting credentials.

To top it off, rye has impressive low glycaemic index credentials, making it a food that helps keep energy levels on an even keel, promoting a sense of satiety and curbing hunger pangs, whilst potentially playing a role in the prevention and management of type II diabetes.

## How to buy it

Experiment and I reckon you'll soon find a loaf you like.

## How to cook it

Rye bread needs an all-action filling, and for that reason single-slice open sandwiches or toast work really well.

## Sun-dried tomato and goat's cheese open sandwich

This offers a welcome break from the boring shop-bought sandwich.

### Serves 1

20 g (¾ oz) sun-dried tomatoes, re-hydrated and roughly chopped
½ garlic clove, crushed
2 tbsp olive oil
8 fresh basil leaves
2 slices wholegrain rye bread
20 g (¾ oz) rocket (arugula)
75 g (2½ oz) soft goat's cheese
Black pepper

Blend the sun-dried tomatoes with the garlic, olive oil and basil to form a paste (I find an electric grinder perfect for this) ■ Generously spread the tomato pesto on to one side of each slice of the rye bread ■ Add a layer of rocket to each, then carefully break the goat's cheese up and arrange on top ■ Season with black pepper.

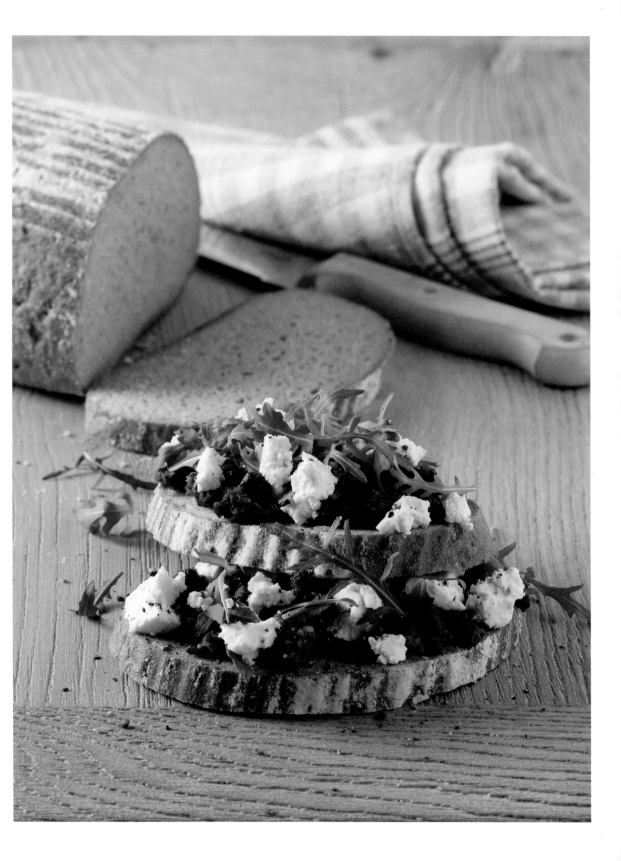

# Strapped for cash

Most of us have been there at one time or another. You know the score. Last month's wages are long gone and you're counting down to pay day, and that generally means one thing – it's time to tighten the purse strings and embark on some serious economizing. And all too often when it comes to food, that means compromising on quality. But is that inevitable? I think not. In fact, I'd stick my neck out and say that the very idea that healthy food has to be expensive is just plain wrong.

Sure, subsisting on a diet of wild salmon, single estate olive oil and wild-crafted goji berries will put a sizeable dent in your pocket. But with a bit of know-how, you can dine in almost as much style, at a fraction of the price. And that involves making the best use of basic staples such as beans and lentils, some choice tinned goods, the best of the locally grown veg that's around and even stuff tucked away in the freezer that you'd probably forgotten was ever there. I reckon it's more than possible to stretch a little bit a long way and see you through to pay day in style.

It's probably no coincidence that some of my best creations in the kitchen have happened with the discovery of an empty fridge (okay, some of my worst, too!). It gets me out of the rut of cooking the same old thing and makes me a whole lot more creative. Mostly it results in a new dish being added to the repertoire, and that's got to be better than giving in and getting a take-away.

If you need more persuading, then I really should mention my mate Matt and his 'Cowboy Pie'. The stuff of legend, it's made literally from what's left in the cupboards (which means no two Cowboy Pies will ever be the same). Living proof that something can always be made from nothing!

# Leeks

I reckon leeks are a bit of an unsung hero. Time to unleash the leek!

## Why you should be eating it

Hailing from the allium family of vegetables, leeks contain appreciable amounts of organosulphur compounds, and eating plenty of this family of foods (which also includes onions and garlic) appears to be related to a reduced risk of stomach cancer.

Judging by all those TV ads for yoghurt drinks containing 'friendly' bacteria, my guess is you know all about probiotics already, but probably a lot less about prebiotics, a type of fibre that stimulates the growth of the good bugs that populate the digestive system. Leeks contain prebiotics in abundance. And not only does this spell happy days for digestive health, but prebiotics also appear to help with absorbing minerals (such as calcium) from our food, and even enhance the way our immune system functions.

Just for good measure, leeks also pack appreciable amounts of carotenoids (notably the eye-friendly lutein and zeaxanthin), antioxidant vitamin C and homocysteine-lowering vitamins B6 and folate.

## How to buy it

Here's my criteria for selecting great leeks and other veg:

1. Ultra fresh
2. Locally grown
3. Seasonal
4. Organic

Tick as many boxes as you can.

## How to cook it

Steam, sautée, braise or slow-cook in hearty soups and casseroles.

## Leek and mustard mash

This has got to be comfort food at its best. It's the food equivalent of getting your duvet down and cozying up on the sofa in front of the television.

### Serves 4

1 kg (2¼ lbs) floury potatoes (such as Maris Piper or King Edward), peeled and chopped into chunks
2 tbsp olive oil
200 g (7 oz) leeks, washed and finely shredded
50 g (1½ oz) butter
4 tbsp milk
2 tbsp wholegrain mustard
Sea salt and black pepper

Place the potatoes in to a large saucepan, cover with cold water, bring to the boil and cook for 20 minutes ■ Meanwhile, heat the olive oil in a frying pan and gently cook the leeks for 10 minutes, or until soft ■ When the potatoes are ready, drain them and return to the saucepan with the butter, milk and mustard. Mash until smooth and creamy. Stir in the leeks, season and serve.

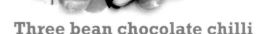

# Beans

When it comes to protein, we tend to think of stuff that comes from animals. As for beans, well they're just seen as a poor man's substitute. But taking a blinkered view like that risks missing out on some hefty goodness.

## Why you should be eating it

Beans are high in protein, low in fat, and a rich source of dietary fibre. That makes them very different to animal protein, which comes with varying amounts of saturated fats, and none of the fibre. Beans are a perfect example of a heart-friendly food, with frequent consumption likely to play a part in helping to reduce levels of 'bad' LDL cholesterol, along with reducing the risk of heart disease and diabetes.

Beans are also a perfect example of a slow-releasing energy food boasting an impressively low glycaemic index. That spells good news for maintaining even energy levels throughout the day and suppressing hunger pangs.

Beans have got other good things going on, too, providing a complex mixture of other nutritional components. These include resistant starch, which acts like a type of food for our friendly gut bacteria, that in turn produce a range of substances beneficial for a healthy digestive system. All in all, looks like poor man's protein has riches aplenty.

## How to buy it

When it comes to beans, I'm more than happy to cheat and get them in a can, opting for the ones without added salt or sugar. But I've always got a stash of dried beans for the times I'm organized enough to do the pre-soaking and cooking from scratch, and I reckon I can taste the difference.

## How to cook it

Being really versatile, I'd happily toss them into soups, casseroles, a chilli or salad.

## Three bean chocolate chilli

You won't even know the minced beef isn't there. Honest.

Serves 4

2 tbsp extra virgin olive oil
1 large onion, finely chopped
2 garlic cloves, crushed
1 celery stick, finely chopped
2 red chillies, deseeded and finely chopped
1 tsp dried oregano
2 tsp ground cumin
¼ tsp ground cinnamon
1 pinch of ground cloves
1 tsp ground coriander
½ tsp chilli powder
1 red and 1 yellow (bell) pepper,
    chopped into small chunks
2 cans mixed beans drained and rinsed
1 can chopped tomatoes
Juice of 1 lime
1 tbsp tamari soy sauce
Black pepper
20 g (¾ oz) dark (semisweet) chocolate
    (70% cocoa solids)
Grated pecorino cheese and/or guacamole
    (see page 108)

Heat the olive oil in a large pan, add the onions and garlic and sauté for 5-10 minutes until the onions are translucent ■ Add the celery and chilli and continue to sauté for 5 minutes ■ Add the herbs, spices and peppers. Stir well and continue to cook for a minute or so. Add a splash of water to prevent the pan from getting too dry. Cover and cook for 5 minutes ■ Add the mixed beans to the pan along with the chopped tomatoes and lime juice ■ Add the tamari soy sauce and black pepper ■ Cover and gently simmer for 10 minutes, stirring occasionally ■ Add the chocolate, let it melt, stir well and serve topped with grated pecorino cheese or guacamole.

# Peas

We used to have great fun as kids shelling peas for Sunday lunch, with a substantial percentage getting devoured without a trace en route to the colander. If I'd known back then they were actually good for me, I reckon it'd have lost its appeal pretty quick.

### Why you should be eating it

It might be a surprise to learn that peas are a decent source of protein, making them an especially good food for vegetarians, or anyone wanting to cut down a tad on their meat intake. And they're quite the crowd pleaser when it comes to their nutritional qualities, containing impressive amounts of homocysteine-lowering folate, the eye protective carotenoids lutein and zeaxanthin, and antioxidant vitamin C. Impressed?

As they're a pulse, peas come with all the benefits they bring to the table, too, such as being packed full of fibre that keeps the digestive system ticking along, whilst offering a helping hand in reducing cholesterol levels and protecting against heart disease.

### How to buy it

Peas are one of the few veg that I nearly always buy frozen. They taste great, retain their goodness and are ridiculously quick to cook. That's not to knock the fresh ones – bang in season and super fresh – they're insanely good.

### How to cook it

I'm not sure that the fish 'n' chip shop mushy peas I grew up with do them any favours, but making your own home-made version is well worth a few minutes labour in the kitchen. They also make for a mean addition to a stir-fry, and if ultra-fresh, are the business when added to salads. And if that's all too much like hard work, then plain and simple boiled (with a sprig of mint if you're feeling flash) served with a knob of butter will do just fine.

## Mushy pesto peas

As much as I like home-made minty mushy peas, this has got an altogether different vibe. I've no problem with convenience, so for this recipe I'd happily use a decent quality pre-made pesto from a jar. But if you want to have a bash at making pesto from scratch (which does taste luscious), I've included a simple recipe on page 71.

### Serves 2

300 g (10½ oz) frozen peas
2 tbsp pesto (see page 71)
2 tbsp extra virgin olive oil
Sea salt and black pepper

Boil the peas in a saucepan for 5 minutes or until cooked ▣ Drain and return to the saucepan (now off the heat) ▣ Add the pesto, olive oil, sea salt and black pepper and get stuck in with a potato masher. Don't be tempted to cheat like my mate Adam did and use a blender – you'll end up with something that resembles baby food ▣ This makes a change from the same old tired veg side dish of boiled broccoli and carrots and would go great with a lovely bit of grilled white fish and some sweet potato chips.

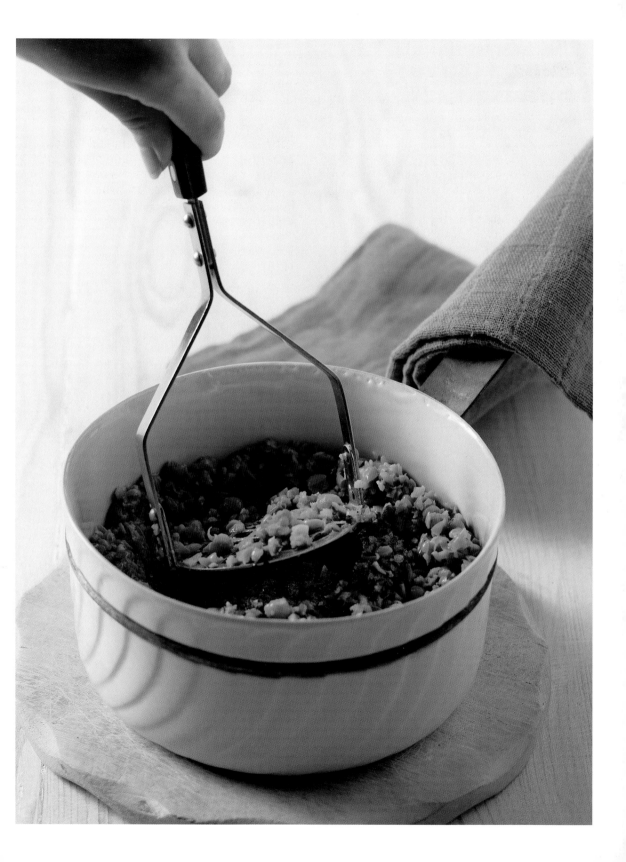

# Broad (Fava) beans

So you don't think broad beans (also known as fava beans) are big time? Well they've broken into Hollywood for a start, courtesy of the villainous Hannibal Lecter ("I ate his liver with some fava beans and a nice chianti"). Okay...

### Why you should be eating it

Broad beans offer a good source of protein, making them an excellent inclusion in vegetarian diets. That's not to say meat eaters don't stand to benefit either. A bit more in the way of vegetarian protein, in place of animal protein, wouldn't go amiss, as it comes minus the saturated fats. (I still reckon ol' Lecter would need some convincing...).

They're also chock-full of dietary fibre, something most of us simply don't get enough of. Not only does this assist in keeping the digestive system ticking along and help reduce the risk of colon cancer, the type of fibre found in pulses aids in lowering cholesterol levels in the blood, spelling good news for heart health, too. A serving of pulses such as broad beans can also count as one of the 'at least 5-a-day' fruit and veg. Bonus.

A note of caution, people with 'favism', an inherited condition in which a protein that helps protect red blood cells from damage is lacking (glucose-6-phosphate dehydrogenase or G6PD), can have a nasty reaction to broad beans and get seriously ill, so should avoid them.

### How to buy it

Broad beans are hardy and easy to grow, making them a favourite of the home-grown veggie patch. As they rapidly lose their flavour, heading for a local farm shop or farmer's market for stuff straight off the field is a good bet. Frozen broad beans are a top-notch substitute.

### How to cook it

Broad beans need to be removed from their pods. Older, larger, tougher beans may also need to be skinned. Broad beans can be transformed into dips, pâté or mash, added to risottos, stews, soups, and pasta dishes.

# Pearl barley risotto with broad beans and mint

A meal on the cheap it might be, but this dish is quite the sophisticate.

### Serves 4

25 g (1 oz) unsalted butter
1 tbsp extra virgin olive oil
1 medium sized onion, finely chopped
300 g (11 oz) pearl barley
1 glass of white wine
1 litre (2 pts) hot vegetable stock
400 g (14 oz) frozen broad (fava) beans

**TO SERVE**
50 g (2 oz) Parmesan cheese, grated
Knob of unsalted butter
Small handful of chopped fresh mint
Zest of 1 unwaxed lemon
Black pepper

Melt the butter in a pan over a low heat, add the olive oil and fry the chopped onion until soft. Add the pearl barley and cook, stirring, for a minute or so. Pour in the white wine and bring to a vigorous boil for a couple of minutes to reduce ■ Pour in half the hot stock and simmer over a gentle heat, stirring to prevent it sticking to the bottom of the pan. Cook for 10 minutes while keeping the remaining stock hot ■ Add the frozen broad beans and a couple of ladles of stock. Raise the heat so that it comes up to the boil quickly and simmer. As the stock is absorbed, add a few more ladles. It should take another 15 minutes ■ Once the beans and pearl barley are cooked, but still with a little bite, turn off the heat and stir through the cheese, knob of butter, mint, lemon zest and black pepper and leave to stand for 5 minutes before serving.

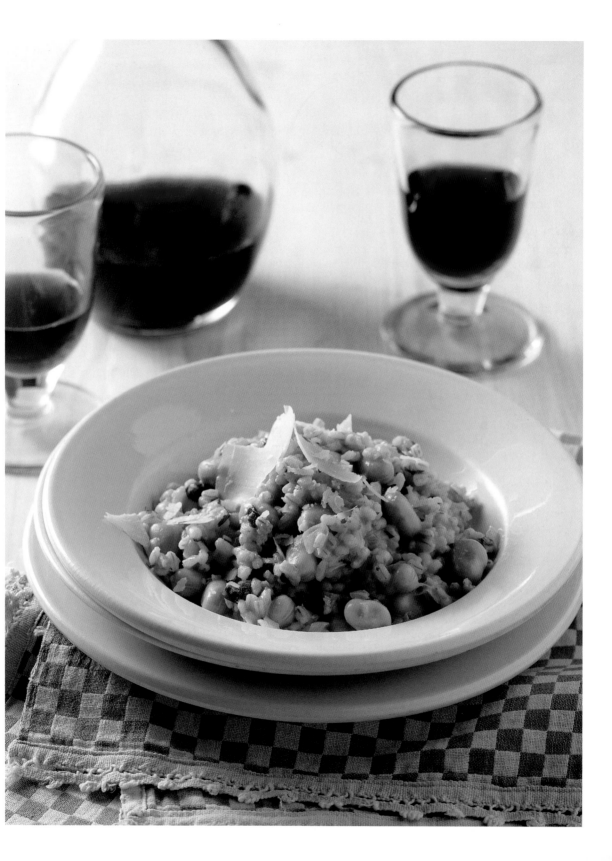

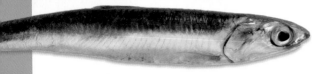

# Anchovies

Being an oily fish, anchovies are a good example of healthy food on the cheap, and having a few jars or cans stashed away is never a bad idea.

## Why you should be eating it

There's loads to be said about oily fish so here we'll take a look at the nutrient content of oily fish, but if you're interested in benefits for heart health, check out mackerel on page 56, for the brain and mood, check out sardines on page 58, or for inflammatory health problems, check out salmon on page 78.

Just like meat, oily fish is an excellent source of protein. But unlike just about any other food, it provides high levels of omega-3 fats in the form of EPA and DHA – and there's a load more about that elsewhere in the book. But oily fish isn't just a one-trick pony, boasting an impressive array of other nutrients, such as fat soluble vitamins A and D, vitamin B12 and the minerals selenium and iodine. Plus if you eat the soft-bones in tinned fish such as sardines, you also get a good dose of calcium.

Vitamin D definitely merits some extra air time, with oily fish being one of the very few foods to contain meaningful amounts. Most of our vitamin D actually comes from exposing the skin to sunshine, which triggers its production. But there are big concerns that many of us aren't getting anywhere near enough vitamin D to stay healthy, which may be putting us at increased risk of a whole string of health problems such as osteoporosis, common cancers, autoimmune diseases, heart disease, even depression.

### EATING OILY FISH

Oily fish have the potential to accumulate various pollutants such as polychlorinated biphenyls (PCBs) and dioxins. To ensure the benefits of eating oily fish, of which there are many, outweigh potential risks, it is recommended that women who are pregnant or breastfeeding, or girls and women who may become pregnant at some point in their lives, should avoid eating more than two portions of oily fish per week. For everyone else, eating up to four portions of oily fish per week is unlikely to pose a problem.

## How to buy it

Typically, anchovies come with a lot of added salt, which is strongly linked with high blood pressure, so should be used only sparingly in recipes. But it's perfectly possible to buy more artisan anchovies, packed in good-quality olive oil, making for an all in all healthier option. Sustainably sourced anchovies are now also more widely available, too.

## How to cook it

Whilst anchovies can be predictably found atop many pizzas they're also great in pasta dishes and salads (Salade Nicoise being a classic example), and their indomitable flavour adds some serious clout to meat, fish and vegetable dishes, and sauces. Capers and olives make for good buddies.

## Pasta with sardines, anchovy and chilli

I knew there had to be more to tinned sardines than sticking them on a bit of toast.

Serves 4

400 g (14 oz) wholewheat spaghetti
4 tbsp extra virgin olive oil
8 anchovy fillets, chopped
2 x 120 g (4 oz) tins of sardines in olive oil, drained and flaked
2 garlic cloves, finely chopped
1 medium red chilli, deseeded and finely chopped
1 x 400 g (14 oz) tin of tomatoes, whizzed in a blender until smooth
Zest and juice of an unwaxed lemon
2 tbsp chopped parsley
Knob of unsalted butter
Black pepper

Bring a large pan of water to the boil and cook the spaghetti until 'al dente' (it should take about 10 minutes) ■ Meanwhile place the oil, chopped anchovies, flaked sardines, chopped garlic and chilli, tomatoes, and the zest and juice of the lemon into a large high-sided frying pan. Cook over a medium heat, stirring occasionally until the sauce has thickened. The sauce should take about as long as it takes for the pasta to cook ■ Once the sauce is ready, stir in the parsley, butter and add pepper to taste ■ Drain the pasta and stir the sauce through so that each strand is well coated. Serve.

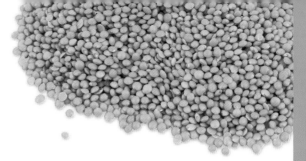

# Red lentils

I disagree with people who think that a meal isn't a meal without a slab of meat on the plate. As well as forming the basis for a hearty dish, simple peasant fare like lentils offer a great way to keep the weekly food bill down.

## Why you should be eating it

The nutritional value of lentils gives meat a run for its money, and in many ways lentils come out on top. Whilst providing a good source of protein, lentils, unlike meat, are full of fibre, with all the benefits that entails for digestive health, along with soluble fibre's cholesterol-lowering properties. And that's definitely not something meat can boast, often containing significant amounts of cholesterol-raising saturated fat.

We tend to think of vegetarians as an anaemic bunch, but the reality is that foodstuff such as lentils contains meaningful amounts of iron. Whilst this isn't in the same highly absorbable form as red meat, having a vitamin C-rich food such as red peppers, tomatoes, green leafy veg, or orange juice at the same time will enhance the uptake.

Lentils are a prime example of a low GI, slow-releasing energy food. The type of food that keeps energy levels on an even keel, helping us feel fuller for longer, thereby aiding weight control. The bottom line is simple. Most of us would be a whole lot healthier if we ate more plant-based food and not too much meat. We'd save a few quid along the way, too.

## How to buy it

Red split lentils are cheap, cheerful and widely available.

## How to cook it

Less fiddly than dried beans, you don't need to spend ages pre-soaking and cooking them. They cook relatively quickly, making them ideal for thickening and filling out soups, casseroles, and my absolute fave, a lovely spicy lentil dhal.

## Vegetable dhal

Not only are the lentils a cheap staple for this dish, but it's also a chance to finally use up the last of the remaining veggies that have been knockin' around in the fridge.

Serves 4

250 g (9 oz) red lentils
1 bay leaf
1 onion, finely chopped
2 garlic cloves, crushed
2 sticks of celery, finely chopped
1 tsp ground cumin
¼ tsp chilli powder
½ tsp grated fresh root ginger
1 tsp turmeric
1 tbsp extra virgin olive oil
250 g (8 oz) mixed vegetables (such as peas, French (green) beans, carrots, spinach), chopped
2 tsp lemon juice
15 g (1 oz) creamed coconut
Black pepper
1 tsp garam masala
2 hard-boiled eggs (optional)
1 onion, chopped and fried (optional)

Place the lentils in a large saucepan with 600 ml (1 pint) of water. Bring to the boil and remove any foam that forms at the edges. Add the bay leaf, half the onion, garlic, celery, cumin, chilli, ginger and turmeric. Cook slowly for approximately 40 minutes until the lentils have collapsed and form a smooth soup-like consistency. Add a little more water if it looks too dry ■ Meanwhile heat the oil in a pan and fry the remaining onion till golden. Add the mixed vegetables. Cover and sweat gently till tender ■ Add the cooked vegetables to the lentil mixture. Stir in the lemon juice, creamed coconut, pepper and garam masala ■ Turn off the heat and leave to stand, covered for 10 minutes ■ Serve over brown rice, and top with the onion and egg, if liked.

# Prawns (Shrimp)

I love a food with a story to tell. Better still if it's got a twist in its tale. Sitting comfortably? Then I'll begin.

## Why you should be eating it

*The opening:* Prawns are laden with cholesterol. Shock, horror, panic.

*The plot unfolds:* But don't let that put you off. In otherwise healthy people, moderate amounts of cholesterol from foods such as prawns don't have a particularly negative impact, if any at all, on cholesterol levels in the blood.

*The twist:* It's actually a diet high in saturated fats, not cholesterol, that's far more likely to push up cholesterol levels. And lo and behold, prawns are low in saturated fat.

*The happy ending:* Prawns also contain a snazzy array of nutrients that might even be touted as 'heart-friendly'. These include a smidgen of cardio-protective omega-3 fats, homocysteine-lowering vitamin B12, and the trace mineral selenium, which can be in short supply.

## How to buy it

When I'm buying prawns, the big dilemma is whether to go shell-on or peeled. Peeling prawns is a bit of a chore, but I reckon they taste loads better. But if time is tight, peeled will do just fine.

## How to cook it

Prawns cook pretty quick, so the trick is to cook them thoroughly without over-cooking. There are loads of good things to do with prawns. A home-made curry is my absolute fave, but prawns are also great in stir-fries and salads, or just served as they are with a lip-smacking dip.

## Prawn and veg curry

If there's one food above all others that I wouldn't be without, it'd be a toss-up between chocolate and curry. Curry would probably win. Just.

### Serves 2

2 tbsp extra virgin olive oil
1 large onion, one half finely chopped and the other half roughly chopped
1 heaped tsp cumin seeds
1 heaped tsp coriander seeds
10 black peppercorns
1 level tsp turmeric powder
¾ tsp black mustard seeds
1 deseeded red chilli, roughly chopped
2 garlic cloves, crushed
100 g (3½ oz) block of creamed coconut, roughly chopped
400 ml (14 fl oz) water
1 red & 1 green (bell) pepper, deseeded and cut into chunks
1 courgette (zucchini), sliced
250 g (9 oz) prawns (shrimp), cooked and peeled
Sea salt

Heat the olive oil in a large pan and gently fry the finely chopped onion for about 5 minutes until translucent ■ Put all of the spices, chilli, garlic, roughly chopped onion, coconut and 300 ml (½ pint) of the water in a blender and blend until really smooth ■ Add the spice mixture to the pan, bring to the boil and simmer for 10 minutes. Stir regularly ■ Add the remaining water and vegetables and bring to the boil. Reduce heat, cover and gently simmer for 20 minutes, stirring occasionally ■ Add the prawns and sea salt to taste. Continue to cook for 4-5 minutes, making sure that the prawns are thoroughly heated through ■ Serve with brown basmati rice or Bombay potatoes.

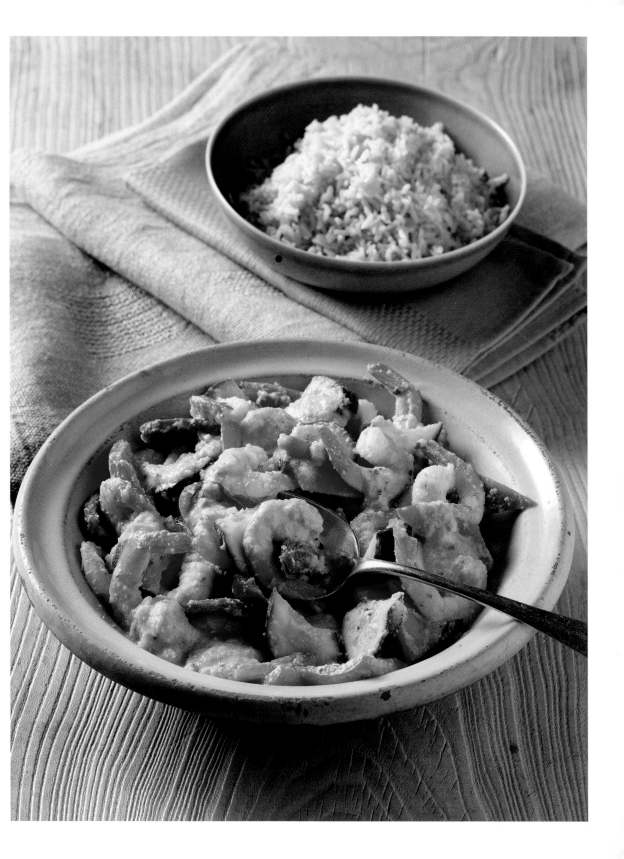

# Summer living

I've no idea what it is about summer that makes food eaten outside taste so much better. Obviously a bit of sunshine goes a long way, and so does the fact that eating outdoors usually involves friends and preferably lots of them. But whatever it is, it most definitely rocks! It's just about the only reason I can come up with to justify a whole chapter in this book. And why not, I say, food's there to be enjoyed after all.

This chapter also sets out to deal in no uncertain terms with two stereotypes that totally depress me. Number one on my hit list is the barbecue. I reckon the all too typical barbecue fare of unidentifiable blackened hunks of meats stuffed inside a sorry looking white bun (probably the tomato ketchup is the healthiest bit!) deserves a well-earned makeover. Number two on my hit list are salads. I want to know how a salad turned out to be a miserable mix-up of limp lettuce, dried out slithers of cucumber, a few slices of insipid tomato, and if you're lucky, a daring sprinkle of cress? All without a dressing! It's no wonder that we can't get people to eat their veg anymore.

It goes without saying that summer is also a time to make the very most of the abundance of lovely fresh, local, seasonal produce that's in plentiful supply. I won't bang on about it too much, I'm sure you've heard it all before, other than to say that the locally grown seasonal stuff tends to be fresher than its imported counterpart. And if it's that much fresher, chances are it'll be more nutritious, and just as importantly, taste a whole lot better to boot. You might even try your hand at growing your own, in which case you'll be unstoppable come summer time!

# Basil

Whilst fruits and vegetables rightly steal the lion's share of the health plaudits, culinary herbs and spices deserve a mention, too.

### Why you should be eating it

A bit like green leafy vegetables but in much smaller doses, basil provides useful amounts of vitamin K, important for strong bones, along with the naturally occurring eye-friendly plant pigments lutein and zeaxanthin.

But it doesn't end there. Lots of herbs and spices have been shown to contain appreciable amounts of potentially health-giving polyphenolic compounds. And this is true for basil. For example, it contains plentiful amounts of rosmarinic acid, which possesses antioxidant and anti-inflammatory properties. And if you opt for the less common purple basil, you're likely to take on board a dose of anthocyanins, too, the same plant pigments responsible for the colour of berries and red grapes, and also possibly some of their health benefits.

That's not to say there's anything particularly special about basil or that we should go out and eat a load of it. There isn't and we shouldn't. But the point it does highlight is the potential benefits to be gained by eating more plant foods, including adding a bit of gastronomic zing with some well chosen culinary herbs and spices. But who am I kidding? The main reason for including basil in the diet is it tastes awesome. And who can argue with that?

### How to buy it

Fresh basil is widely available and at its tastiest plucked straight from the plant and used right away. So if you've got a space on your kitchen windowsill, make good use of it.

### How to cook it

Fresh basil can be added to summer salads, especially those involving tomatoes. It's a great addition to tomato sauces or pasta dishes, either shredded or in the form of a corker of a fresh pesto.

## Tomato, mozzarella and basil salad

This is a classic, and makes a simple starter or light summer salad. For this to work well you need some properly ripe tomatoes. If you can beg, borrow or steal some home-grown ones for this, do it. If not, vine-ripened tomatoes should do the trick.

**Serves 4 as a main course or 8 as a starter**

8 ripe medium tomatoes
4 buffalo mozzarella (about 400-500 g/1 lb in total)
1 small bunch fresh basil
4 tbsp extra virgin olive oil
Black pepper

Thinly slice the tomatoes and arrange them on a large plate or platter ■ Slice the mozzarella and arrange on top of the tomatoes ■ Roughly shred or tear the basil leaves and scatter on top of the mozzarella ■ Generously drizzle with olive oil and season with black pepper.

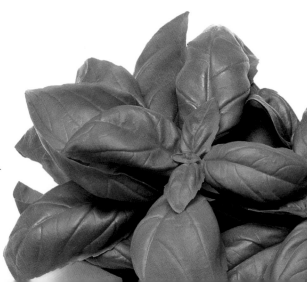

# Rocket (Arugula)

I always feel as though I've gone a bit posh when I add rocket to a salad, but it really does taste good.

## Why you should be eating it

Like many of the green leafy veg, rocket is laden with such noteworthy bone-building nutrients as calcium and magnesium, bolstered by a decent bit of vitamin K. And true to form for a green leafy veg, it also provides a plentiful supply of folate.

Rocket also offers up a choice range of antioxidants and phytochemicals, notably satisfying levels of vitamin C and carotenoids. Of the carotenoids, rocket is especially abundant in lutein and zeaxanthin, a high dietary intake of which looks likely to keep eyes healthy with advancing years, notably being associated with protection against age-related macular degeneration and cataracts.

It may come as a surprise that rocket is actually a cruciferous vegetable (other cruciferous veggies include cabbage, watercress, broccoli and Brussels sprouts) and as such contains a uniquely rich source of glucosinolates (notably glucoraphanin), the compounds that give rocket its peppery taste. These get converted to bio-active isothiocyanates when we eat them, which are thought to proffer cancer protective properties.

## How to buy it

You can happily pick up bags of fresh rocket from just about any supermarket, or you could have a go at growing your own.

## How to cook it

Rocket is a sure-fire way to add a peppery twist to all-too-frequent drab mixed salads. Another good bet is to make a fresh rocket pesto. It can also be added to soups, stews or pasta dishes towards the end of cooking.

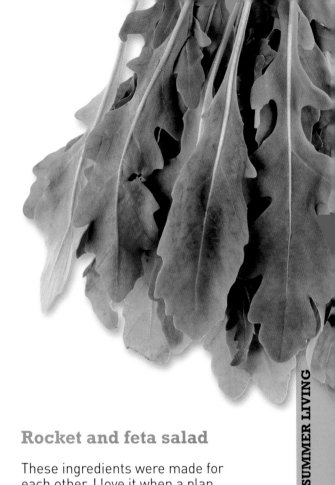

## Rocket and feta salad

These ingredients were made for each other. I love it when a plan comes together...

Serves 4

100 g (4 oz) rocket (arugula)
200 g (7 oz) feta, cubed
150 g (5 oz) cherry tomatoes, halved
200 g (7 oz) frozen peas, defrosted

FOR THE DRESSING
6 tbsp extra virgin olive oil
2 tbsp lemon juice
2 tbsp white wine vinegar
Black pepper

Mix all the salad ingredients together in a serving bowl ■ Whisk together all the ingredients for the dressing and pour over the salad. Toss gently and serve.

# Mackerel

Mackerel has got to be one of the most underrated foods going, but bought fresh and cooked well, it tastes amazing.

## Why you should be eating it

Here we're shining a spotlight on the benefits of oily fish for heart health. If you want more on its general nutritional value check out anchovies on page 48, for a low-down on its reputation as brain-food head to sardines on page 58, or for its anti-inflammatory benefits, flip to salmon on page 78.

Researchers first got interested in the benefits of oily fish in reducing the risk of heart disease with the discovery that Eskimos in Greenland, with a diet high in omega-3 fats (including from whale blubber and seal fat, yum), had a strikingly low rate of deaths from coronary heart disease. Ever since, researchers have been clammering to get to the bottom of the omega-3 story.

The cardio-protective effect of omega-3 fats from oily fish looks likely to be due to a number of different mechanisms, working together. Whilst they have little effect on cholesterol levels they appear to lower levels of triglycerides (a type of fat) in the blood, help to prevent the blood from clotting, exert a positive effect on blood pressure, help regulate the rhythm of the heart beat and assist in keeping the lining of blood vessels healthy and working well.

Here's the bottom line: omega-3 fish oils appear to reduce the chance of having a fatal heart attack. Considering that cardiovascular disease is the leading cause of death in many Western countries, regular inclusion of oily fish once, maybe twice a week, sounds like a pretty useful prescription for good health.

## How to buy it

As with all fish, the key is to get it as ultra fresh as possible. And think sustainability by choosing fish certified by the Marine Stewardship Council (MSC).

## How to cook it

Grilling and barbecuing are my personal favourites, baking coming a close second. And don't forget mackerel pâté.

## Barbecued mackerel with orange salsa

I'm all for making life easier, so I'd definitely recommend one of those hinged wire fish rack thingies for cooking whole fish on the barbie.

### Serves 2

2 mackerel, cleaned and gutted but left whole
Extra virgin olive oil

FOR THE SALSA
2 large oranges
½ red onion, sliced thinly
Medium handful of fresh coriander (cilantro), roughly chopped
100 g (3½ oz) pitted black olives, halved
1 tbsp extra virgin olive oil

First up, the salsa. Slice the top and bottom off each orange so that it stands steady on the chopping board. Take a small knife and cut away the peel and pith so that you're just left with the orange flesh. Halve each orange, halve again and cut into slices ■ Place the orange slices into a serving bowl and toss with the remaining salsa ingredients. Leave to stand at room temperature for up to an hour so the flavours amalgamate ■ When the barbecue is ready to roll, take each fish and make a couple of deep slashes along its side. Brush each side with olive oil. Place them in a wire grilling basket and barbecue till done ■ Once the fish are cooked, serve immediately with the orange salsa and some crusty bread to mop the juices.

### ◄ EATING OILY FISH

Oily fish have the potential to accumulate various pollutants such as polychlorinated biphenyls (PCBs) and dioxins. To ensure the benefits of eating oily fish, of which there are many, outweigh potential risks, it is recommended that women who are pregnant or breastfeeding, or girls and women who may become pregnant at some point in their lives, should avoid eating more than two portions of oily fish per week. For everyone else, eating up to four portions of oily fish per week is unlikely to pose a problem.

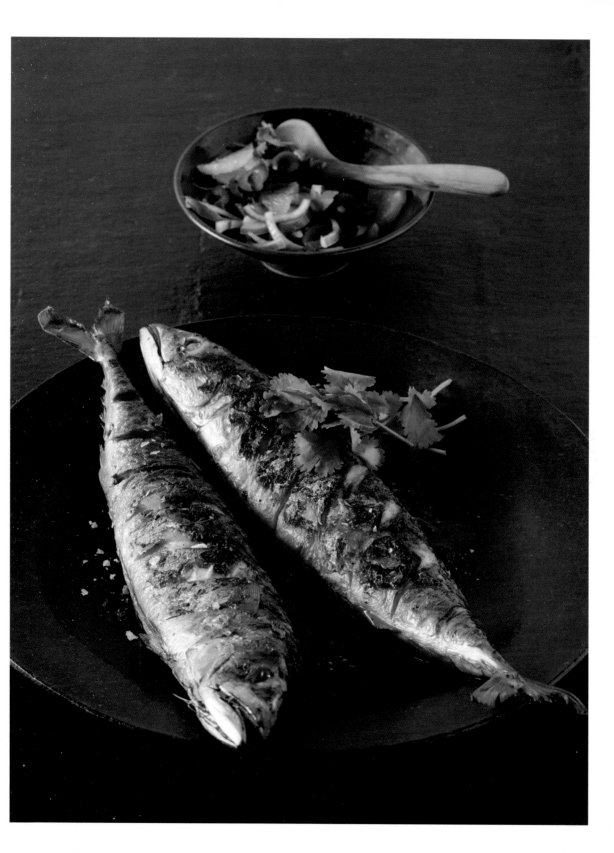

# Sardines

If you thought sardines only came out of a tin, you might be surprised at how different the fresh ones taste.

## Why you should be eating it

Here I'll be taking a close look at whether the old wives tale about fish being brain food has any truth to it. But if you want to know more about the nutritional value of oily fish then take a look at anchovies on page 48, for a low-down on the benefits for heart health, check out mackerel on page 56, and for their effects on inflammatory health problems, suss out salmon on page 78.

Of the two types of omega-3 fats found in oily fish, EPA and DHA, it's the DHA that's important for the structure of the brain. And that explains its important role in aiding the development of young brains, especially during the last trimester of pregnancy and the first couple of years of life.

But omega-3 fats appear to be important for brain function throughout our whole life cycle, not just during infancy. There's a lot of interest in their potential to prevent and improve the symptoms of depression, and possibly other mental health problems, too. They may also have a role to play in helping some children with behavioural and learning problems like dyspraxia, dyslexia and ADHD, and even with helping to keep the brain working well into old age by reducing the risk of dementia and cognitive decline.

### 🐟 EATING OILY FISH

Oily fish have the potential to accumulate various pollutants such as polychlorinated biphenyls (PCBs) and dioxins. To ensure the benefits of eating oily fish, of which there are many, outweigh potential risks, it is recommended that women who are pregnant or breastfeeding, or girls and women who may become pregnant at some point in their lives, should avoid eating more than two portions of oily fish per week. For everyone else, eating up to four portions of oily fish per week is unlikely to pose a problem.

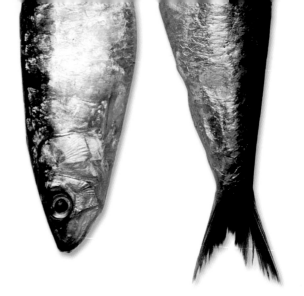

## How to buy it

As with all fish, your mission should be to get it as sparklingly fresh as you possibly can.

## How to cook it

Simply grill, barbecue or bake.

## Grilled sardines with mint, lime and chilli

These are great cooked on the barbecue, wrapped in foil packets to trap all the flavour in.

### Serves 4

Few sprigs of fresh mint, finely chopped
1 red chilli, deseeded and finely chopped
3 garlic cloves, finely chopped
Zest and juice of 2 unwaxed limes
8–12 fresh sardines, cleaned, prepared and ready to cook

Mix the mint, chilli, garlic and lime zest and juice together in a small bowl and push about a teaspoon of the mix into the cavity of each of the fish ■ Fold four large pieces of foil in half and place 2–3 sardines on top of each. Wrap the foil over the fish and seal well ■ Pop on to the barbecue and cook for about 20 minutes, or until cooked through, turning half way ■ To serve, place each parcel onto a plate, allowing each person to open their individual package to get a good hit of the amazing aroma ■ Great served with a simple tomato and garlic salad and some crusty bread.

# Steak

On the whole we should be eating more plant foods and less meat. But if we are to eat red meat, better that we eat it sparingly, go for good-quality lean cuts, and have a greater appreciation of the health benefits, as well as the risks it poses.

## Why you should be eating it

Beef provides an excellent source of protein, the minerals selenium, zinc and iron, along with vitamin B12. Some of the nutrients you'll find in beef, and I'm thinking of the zinc and especially the iron, are really well absorbed compared with plant sources.

Iron in steak comes in the form of 'haem' iron, much easier to absorb than the 'non-haem' iron found in plant foods (although they're still really useful sources of iron, too). One of the most important functions of iron is to form haemoglobin in red blood cells, which play the vital role of transporting oxygen around the body. If iron levels in the body get really low, this leads to anaemia.

But beef loses some brownie points, too. Red meat generally contains appreciable amounts of saturated fat, the type linked with increased cholesterol levels in the blood and heart disease. That would suggest that a nice lean bit of steak is a better option compared with fatty cuts of meat, or processed meat products. Eating a lot of red meat is also linked with increased risk of colon cancer, so easy does it.

## How to buy it

I view steak as a real treat, not an everyday food. And that's why I'll go for a good-quality, preferably organic steak every time.

## How to cook it

We've all got a view on cooking the perfect steak. Just remember that resting it before serving is probably almost as important as the actual cooking itself. And one thing worth knowing is that meat cooked at high temperatures that leads to a charred or burnt effect generates harmful chemicals linked with an increased risk of cancer. I'm not trying to put you off – life's there to be enjoyed after all – but eating charred meat is definitely not something you'd want to make a habit of.

## Spice-rubbed barbecued steak

Whilst we want a good-quality bit of steak to do the talking, this spice rub is the business. Try to remember to take the steak out of the fridge 15 minutes or so before you cook it, just enough time for it to come up to room temperature.

FOR 1 STEAK
1 tsp mixed peppercorns
½ tsp mustard seeds
½ tsp paprika
A little extra virgin olive oil

Bash up the spices in a grinder or pestle and mortar into a coarse powder. Mix in a little olive oil to give a thickish paste ▓ Pour onto the steak and give it a good ol' rub in ▓ Pop it on to the grill and cook to your liking ▓ Once cooked, move the steak on to the side of the grill, away from the main source of heat. Let it rest for a couple of minutes or so. Then it's good to go.

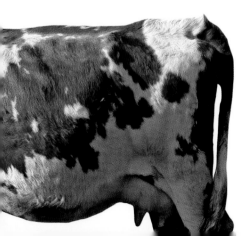

# Halloumi

Okay, I'll be straight with you. I don't think cheese is all that much of an amazingly healthy food. But honestly, can you imagine life without some of those lovely cheeses like mozzarella, feta or halloumi? And that's my point. I reckon enjoying food is really important. There's definitely more to life than just eating ultra-healthy stuff all the time.

## Why you should be eating it

Cheeses such as halloumi have their good points for sure. It comes packed with protein for a start, indispensable for growth and repair. And of course, made from milk, it's also a cracking source of calcium. Not only is this an essential mineral for strong bones, but a calcium-rich diet may have a role to play in helping to reduce body weight and body fat (although low fat dairy products are likely to be a better option when it comes to shedding a few pounds).

Of course, there is the saturated fat to contend with, although halloumi does tend to be lower in fat than most hard cheeses, not to mention the salt. But then you probably knew that already. And at the end of the day, it's a pretty natural, unadulterated food, unlike many of the highly processed, refined, pre-packaged foods that typify modern diets. That's the stuff we should be more worried about.

## How to buy it

Traditionally, halloumi is made from sheep's milk and/or goat's milk, making it an ideal choice for anyone intolerant to cow's milk, but tolerant of other milks. However, it's typical to see cow's milk added to most of the commercially produced halloumi on sale, so if in doubt, check the label.

## How to cook it

Halloumi is generally used as a cooked cheese and is at its best grilled until golden, making it ideal for barbecuing on a skewer.

## Halloumi kebabs

Kebabs don't exactly have a glowing reputation as a health food. But when push comes to shove, it's all about the quality of the ingredients used. And there's nothing stopping you using top drawer ingredients for this.

### Serves 1

2 tbsp extra virgin olive oil
Zest and juice of ½ unwaxed lemon
1 garlic clove, crushed
1 tbsp chopped mixed fresh herbs (such as rosemary, mint, thyme and oregano)
Black pepper

FOR THE KEBABS
6 cherry tomatoes
6 button mushrooms
½ red (bell) pepper, diced into good sized pieces
125 g (4½ oz) halloumi cheese, cubed
You'll need 2 wooden kebab skewers, soaked in cold water for ½ an hour (this will stop them burning on the barbecue)

Mix all of the ingredients for the marinade together in a bowl ▦ Add the prepared vegetables and cheese to the marinade and gently combine so that everything is coated. Leave to marinate for at least 30 minutes ▦ Thread a piece of cheese, pepper, a whole mushroom and tomato onto the skewers and repeat until you have 3 of each on each skewer. Pour any remaining marinade over the kebabs ▦ Grill on the barbecue, turning gently so that they are browned on all sides.

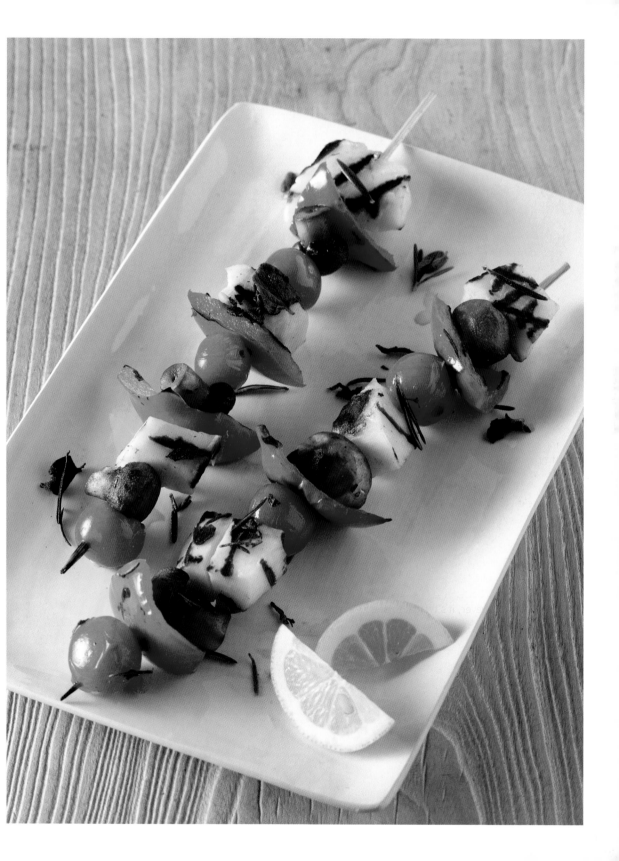

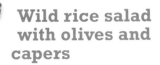

# Parsley

When used well, fresh herbs can make an average dish taste fantastic. And the likes of parsley, which can be used liberally, can do big things for the nutritional value, too.

## Why you should be eating it

Most people struggle to include decent amounts of green leafy veg in their diets. Let's face it, if you want to notch up brownie points by eating something healthy, blueberries are going to win over kale every time. But parsley, being all green and leafy, does contain lots of the same nutrients. And whilst we're not going to eat it in the same quantities as vegetables, at least it's a start.

So in true green leafy style, parsley packs away good levels of antioxidants in the form of vitamin C and carotenoids. Then we have bone-building vitamin K along with a dash of calcium, heart-friendly homocysteine-lowering folate, and a decent bit of iron for good measure.

Just like fruits and veggies, parsley contains an array of health-promoting phytochemicals. One such example is the flavone apigenin. Found in abundance in parsley, researchers have found it to possess impressive anti-inflammatory, anti-oxidant and potential anti-cancer properties. That doesn't mean you should go out and eat loads of parsley, as exactly how normal dietary amounts of these substances affect our health is still relatively unknown. But it does highlight the vast diversity of beneficial plant compounds that are on offer from diets containing a really good variety of fruits, veggies and plant foods.

## How to buy it

Fresh parsley is widely available by the bunch or bag, but if it's maximum freshness you're hankering for then nothing beats the stuff freshly snipped from a pot or the herb garden.

## How to cook it

Used as a garnish for purely decorative means won't reap much in the way of nutrients. To harvest those benefits, I'm up for more generous amounts being used to big-up the flavour of salads, soups, casseroles and sauces.

## Wild rice salad with olives and capers

Cooked rice is one of those foods that can cause an unwelcome bout of food poisoning if it's left hanging around at room temperature for too long. So once you've cooked the rice, make sure you cool it down as quickly as possible (ideally within one hour), preferably by dividing it into smaller portions or spreading it out on a shallow tray. Store in the fridge and eat within one day.

Serves 4

175 g (6 oz) brown basmati rice
100 g (4 oz) wild rice
150 g (5 oz) puy lentils
100 g (4 oz) green olives, halved
3 tbsp capers, rinsed
1 red (bell) pepper, finely diced
150 g (5 oz) cherry tomatoes, halved
Good handful parsley, chopped

FOR THE DRESSING
5 tbsp extra virgin olive oil
2 tbsp lemon juice
2 garlic cloves, crushed
1 tsp Dijon mustard
1 tsp honey
Black pepper

Place both rices into a pan and pour over 800ml (1½ pts) of boiling water. Cover with a tight fitting lid and simmer for approximately 35–40 minutes until the rice is tender and the water has been absorbed ■ Meanwhile cook the lentils in plenty of boiling water for approximately 30 minutes ■ Whilst all that's going on, you've time to make the dressing. Whisk together all the dressing ingredients until creamy ■ When the rice and lentils are cooked, drain off any water and place them both into a serving bowl. Pour over the dressing and mix well. Cool quickly ■ To finish off, mix in the olives, capers, red pepper, tomatoes and parsley. Cover and store in the fridge until required.

# Beetroot (Beet)

As a kid, I remember we used to have those crinkle cut slices that came pickled in jars of vinegar. I'm starting to feel queasy just thinking about it. But I'm a big fan of fresh beetroot, both for its taste and its health credentials.

## Why you should be eating it

Beetroot contains unique antioxidants, notably the betalains, the pigments responsible for beetroots shock red colour, which may offer some protection against the damaging effects of excessive free radicals.

Along with good amounts of fibre and potassium, beetroot offers up plentiful supplies of folate. As well as its importance for mums to be, folate is one of the key nutrients that assist the body in breaking down a substance in the bloodstream called homocysteine, high levels of which are implicated in heart disease and possibly other conditions such as Alzheimer's disease.

Whilst it's unlikely to be top of most people's list of favourite beverages, beetroot juice has squeezed into the spotlight with recent research showing it to have potential blood pressure-lowering qualities.

## How to buy it

In peak condition, beetroots will be really firm to the touch. If they feel at all squishy, or look wrinkly, they've been knocking around too long. In the spirit of celebrating home-grown produce, keep it real by sourcing local, seasonal produce whenever you can.

## How to cook it

Either cooked and sliced, or grated raw, beetroots add a bit of visual showbiz to a salad. And if you've never baked them whole, you should give it a bash. Beetroots can also be used in soups, Borscht being the best-known example.

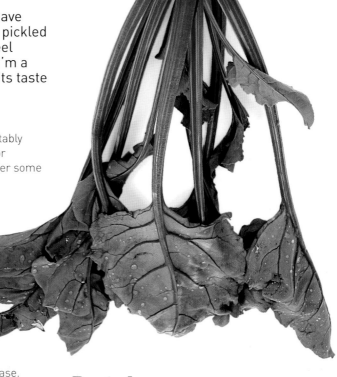

## Beet-slaw

Coleslaw traditionalists, get ready to be horrified. Everyone else, get stuck in.

Serves 4

1 medium sized beetroot (beet), peeled and grated
1 apple, grated
1 large carrot, peeled and grated

FOR THE DRESSING
2 tbsp mayonnaise
2 tbsp natural live yoghurt
1 tbsp balsamic vinegar
1 tsp lemon juice
1 tsp caraway seeds
Black pepper

Combine the beetroot, apple and carrot until evenly mixed ▦ Mix all the dressing ingredients and stir into the beetroot, apple and carrot until thoroughly coated ▦ Chill until ready to serve.

# About oils

I've got no time for extreme, ultra low-fat diets. You've only got to take a look at the Mediterranean diet, one of the healthiest diets around, to see that a moderate intake (of mostly good fats) is no bad thing. And that's the whole point. It's the quality of fats in the diet that counts for a lot.

So whilst we should look to cut back on saturated fats, the type found in fatty cuts of red meats, processed meats, butter, full-fat dairy products, pastries, cakes and the like, and definitely try to avoid the villainous trans fats found in so many of our everyday commercially

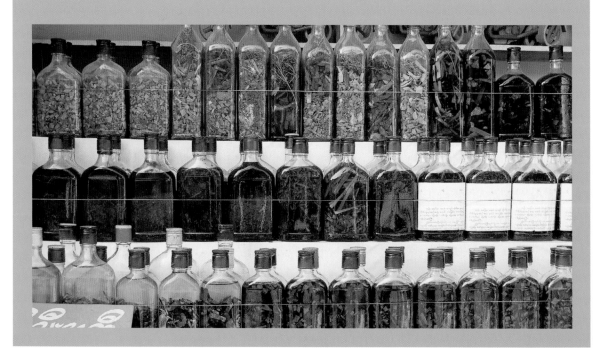

prepared convenience foods, we don't need to skimp on healthy fats. A reasonably low-fat diet, sure, but getting some good fats in the diet is generally to be encouraged.

I'm not averse to using a bit of organic butter in cooking from time to time, it does taste really good after all. But, on the whole, we should be favouring more of the unsaturated fats instead. So here I've selected three examples of healthy oils to think about including in the diet. It's not definitive – there are other healthy oils out there – but these are three that I wouldn't be without.

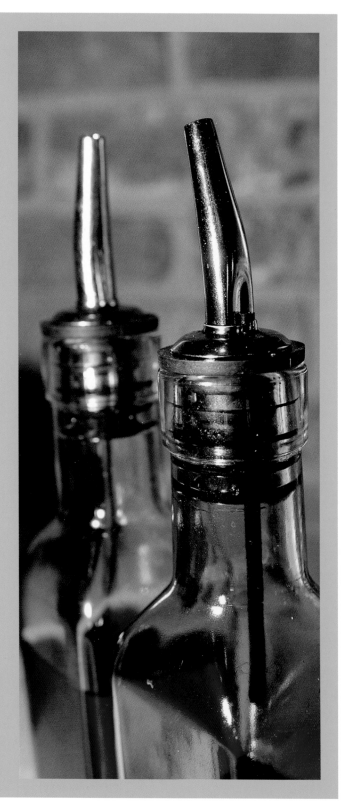

## Olive oil

The cornerstone of the Mediterranean diet, olive oil is a perfect example of a healthful oil. It contains mostly monounsaturated fats, which are generally seen as cardio-protective. This is down to their ability to lower levels of 'bad' LDL cholesterol, whilst at the same time maintaining levels of the 'good' HDL cholesterol. This benefit would be seen most clearly if they replaced some of the saturated fats in the diet.

Generally speaking, I want my oils as unprocessed as possible, so I'd opt for extra virgin olive, which comes from the first cold-pressing of the olives. Better still if it's unfiltered. As well as being big on flavour, it will also preserve a higher level of the naturally occurring beneficial phenolic compounds found in abundance in extra virgin olive oil. These possess antioxidant properties and endow extra virgin olive oil with health benefits beyond that of just being a source of monounsaturated fat.

## Rapeseed oil

I'm not going to repeat myself, suffice to say that rapeseed oil is rich in monounsaturated fats, so we can expect it to mirror similar heart-healthy credentials to olive oil.

What distinguishes rapeseed oil from olive oil is that it contains less saturated fat than olive oil, and significantly higher levels of the beneficial omega-3 fat, alpha-linolenic acid. Because we need this fat to stay healthy, and the body can't make it for itself, we rely on getting it from our diet. That makes it an 'essential fat'. With modern diets tending to contain too much omega-6 fats at the expense of insufficient omega-3 fats, rapeseed oil represents a useful counterbalance.

Personally, I steer clear of the commercially refined rapeseed oils and, just like with olive oil, go for the good-quality, cold-pressed extra virgin stuff that packs maximum flavour and maximum goodness. And because it contains appreciable amounts of fragile omega-3 fats, I'd be avoiding heating this oil to really high temperatures, and be more up for using it for dressings or drizzling.

## Hemp seed oil

Little known outside healthfood circles, cold-pressed hemp seed oil is quite the catch. It provides predominantly healthful polyunsaturated fats, both of the omega-3 and omega-6 kind. And here's the deal breaker. Whilst we need both of those fats in our diets to stay healthy, it's really important to have them in the right balance. And hempseed oil comes up trumps with a pretty ideal balance of both, something not many other oils can boast.

It's also one of the only dietary sources of a specific type of omega-6 fat called gamma-linolenic acid, or GLA, just like the active ingredient in evening primrose oil. This gets converted into hormone-like substances called prostaglandins that regulate lots of important things in the body. Not only does GLA appear to be useful for some women when it comes to promoting healthy hormones (hence the popularity of evening primrose oil amongst PMS sufferers), but it's also good stuff for skin health, and may be useful in conditions such as eczema.

But to preserve those delicate poly-unsaturated fats, which don't like to be exposed to heat, light or oxygen, look for cold-pressed hemp seed oil in a darkened bottle. Once opened, keep it in the fridge. And remember this is definitely not for cooking – we're talking about an oil that you'd use sparingly as a dressing or a drizzler.

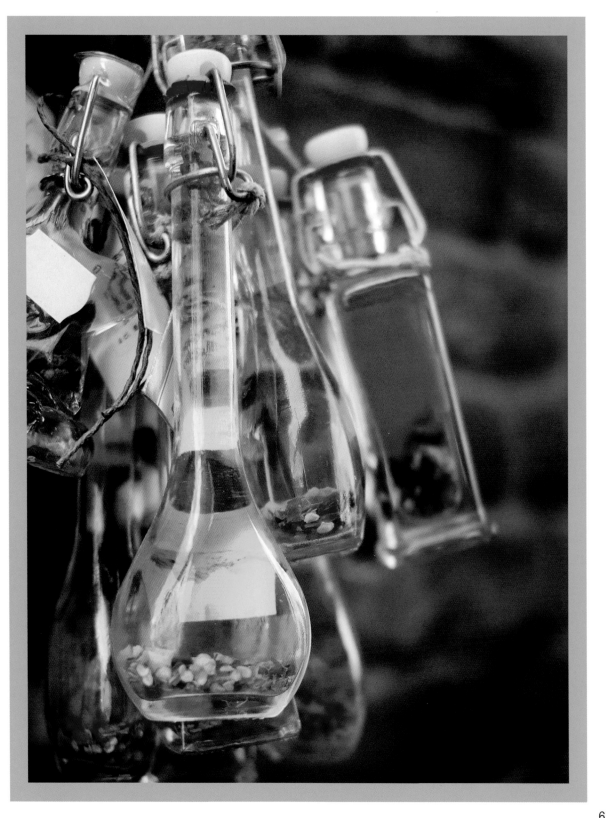

# Lemon

Unless you're into sucking lemons (and I've no idea why you would be!), this is not the sort of food for casual snacking. But when it comes to working some culinary magic, I reckon lemons are pretty much indispensable.

## Why you should be eating it

As with other citrus fruits, lemons provide a bumper crop of vitamin C. Amongst its numerous benefits, vitamin C helps to maintain healthy connective tissue, acts as an anti-oxidant to help protect against the damaging effects of free radicals, and helps increase the absorption of iron from the diet.

Citrus fruits such as lemons are also a rich source of beneficial plant compounds called flavonoids. These are widely distributed in the likes of fruits, vegetables, tea, red wine and cocoa and higher dietary intakes appear to be associated with health benefits, namely a reduced risk of heart disease.

## How to buy it

Look for firm, bright yellow lemons. The ones packing more juice will tend to feel heavier for their size. Lemons that look a bit green are probably under-ripe and will tend to be more acidic. Also citrus fruits are often waxed and you probably don't want to be grating that into your lemon chicken. So if you're planning on using the zest, keep your eyes peeled for the unwaxed versions.

## How to cook it

Salad dressings, marinades, sliced and cooked with fish, stuffed inside a roast chicken, sorbet, home-made lemonade. Loads of possibilities. You get the picture.

## Tahini and lemon dressing

Our fat phobia generally means that dressings get the cold shoulder, but this light and refreshing dressing chalks up some serious brownie points for its nutritional value.

2 tbsp light tahini paste
2 tbsp Greek yoghurt
1 tbsp extra virgin olive oil
Juice of 1 unwaxed lemon
Zest of ½ unwaxed lemon
1 tsp clear honey
4 tbsp water

Mix all of the ingredients except the water together in a bowl until a really even consistency is achieved ▪ Gradually add the water, bit by bit, until you have the desired consistency, which should be perfect for drizzling over a lovely summer salad.

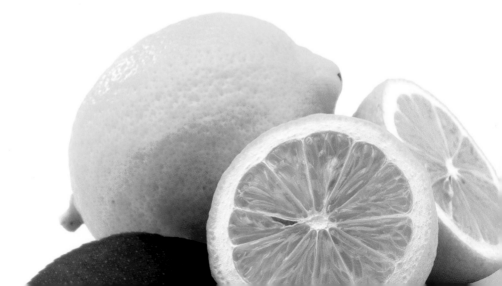

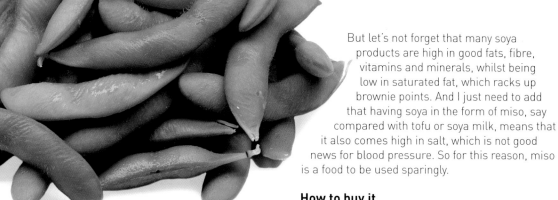

# Miso

Miso is made from fermented soya beans. And soya is one those foods that has managed to generate a right old kerfuffle. Opinion is divided as to whether soya is a good thing or not, and it seems like just about every other person has got their slant on it.

## Why you should be eating it

Soya is a rich source of isoflavones, the main ones being genistein and daidzein. These are known in the game as phytoestrogens – basically plant compounds with weak oestrogenic activity.

Soya beans fell under the glare of the researcher's spotlight when it was discovered that countries with a high intake, like Japan, had relative immunity to some chronic diseases such as breast cancer, compared to countries with a low intake, such as the USA or the UK. Interesting stuff, but of course there're lots of other differences in the diets, lifestyles, even genetics, between these countries, which could be just as important.

So whilst this type of data, what's known as epidemiological evidence, shows that there might be some benefits from lifelong soya intake on reducing breast cancer risk, experimental evidence has not always supported this idea – in fact, some has shown the opposite. The bottom line is that it's a pretty confused picture and the jury is still out on this one.

Other purported health benefits of soya and its isoflavones include positive effects on cardiovascular health, bone health and improving menopausal symptoms, and whilst there is some evidence of benefit in each of these, it's a bit inconsistent.

But let's not forget that many soya products are high in good fats, fibre, vitamins and minerals, whilst being low in saturated fat, which racks up brownie points. And I just need to add that having soya in the form of miso, say compared with tofu or soya milk, means that it also comes high in salt, which is not good news for blood pressure. So for this reason, miso is a food to be used sparingly.

## How to buy it

I reckon the nicest miso pastes are the more authentic, traditionally fermented and aged ones, which you can pick up in good health food shops and most of the bigger supermarkets. There are different varieties of miso, with their own unique taste and personality. But I'm no miso connoisseur – it's hard enough choosing a good bottle of plonk – so I don't get too hung up on the intricacies of it all. Try some different ones, see what you like.

## How to cook it

Miso is most well-known as the integral ingredient in miso soup, but I reckon it can be used in lots of imaginative ways. A good miso paste packs some serious flavour, and a spoonful or two (you don't need much) can readily replace stock cubes and give loads of depth to a hearty soup, casserole, even a rich miso gravy.

## Lime, miso and ginger dressing

With its bold flavours, this is a humdinger of a dressing, guaranteed to add some serious oomph to just about any salad or vegetable dish.

Juice of 1 lime
2 tbsp toasted sesame oil
2 tbsp extra virgin olive oil
1 tsp miso paste
1 tbsp water
1 cm (½ in) fresh root ginger, peeled and finely grated
1 garlic clove, crushed
Small pinch dried chilli flakes

Combine all the ingredients and mix vigorously. Done!

# Chives

Whilst garlic might be the most potent of the allium family, and the most extensively studied for its health benefits, those wanting a milder version might do well to give chives a look-in.

## Why you should be eating it

Like many a culinary herb, chives pack their fair share of vitamins, but as we only eat them in relatively small amounts, it's not really worth writing home about.

Yet chives are a member of the allium family, which also includes the likes of onions and garlic. These allium vegetables are a rich source of flavanols and organosulfur compounds that show anti-cancer effects in lab experiments. Whilst this doesn't prove anything by itself, the idea that allium veggies are a worthy dietary inclusion finds further support from observational studies that associate their consumption with a reduced risk of certain cancers, most notably stomach cancer.

## How to buy it

As a rule of thumb, when it comes to culinary usage, fresh herbs rule over the dried version, and fresh chives should be easy enough to get hold of. Better still, get a mini herb garden on the go – there's nothing quite like snipping off a few fresh herbs for immediate kitchen use.

## How to cook it

Chives, being more mellow than garlic and onions, can be used in many dishes. They're great in omelettes or finely chopped and sprinkled on soups. They also add a bit of interest to salads and taste the business with anything from potatoes to fish.

# Citrus chive dressing

This light and zesty little number will big-up just about any green leafy salad or selection of steamed  greens.

4 tbsp extra virgin cold-pressed rapeseed or olive oil
Juice of 1 lemon
10 g (¼ oz) fresh chives, very finely chopped
1 shallot, very finely chopped
½ tsp Dijon mustard
Sea salt and black pepper

Proper simple. Give all the ingredients a vigorous mix and season with black pepper and a tiny touch of sea salt.

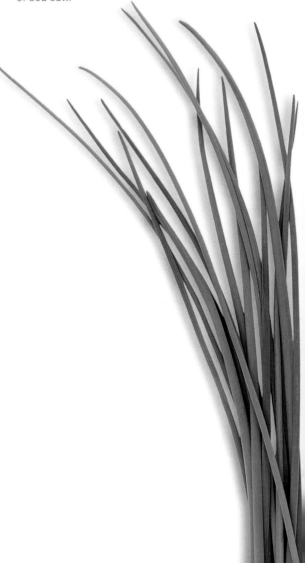

# Pine nuts

I can't really think pine nuts without thinking pesto, so I'm going to take this opportunity for a swift Mediterranean detour.

### Why you should be eating it

There's no denying that pine nuts (they're actually a seed not a nut) are a fully-fledged high fat food. But we really need to fine-tune the way we think about fat and take on board the idea that the quality of fats in our diet, not just the quantity, is important. And just like other nuts and seeds, pine nuts weigh in with mighty amounts of 'good' mono and polyunsaturated fats. And unlike the saturated kind, which raise levels of 'bad' LDL cholesterol and increase the risk of heart disease, these unsaturated fats tend to have the opposite effect.

If you need more convincing then the Mediterranean diet is a fine case in point. First up there's loads more to it than guzzling olive oil, although liberal use of olive oil as the predominant dietary fat is a given. But the Mediterranean diet is also typified by plenty of fruit, veg and cereals, along with fish, legumes and nuts, some wine with meals, and low to moderate amounts of dairy products, poultry and eggs, with even lower amounts of red meat.

All told, it's not a low fat diet, rather a moderate fat diet, but the big difference is that a majority of the fats are of the healthy unsaturated type. And viewed as a whole, it's a dietary pattern associated not only with a reduced risk of heart disease, but potentially favourable effects in the prevention or management of such chronic health problems as cancer, diabetes, obesity and Alzheimer's disease. Oh yeah, and it's a 'diet' that actually tastes good!

### How to buy it

Pine nuts can be pricey little things, so I'd tend to use them in fairly small amounts. Mostly you'll find them shelled and in their raw state. As they're liable to go rancid if left knocking around too long, I'd be looking to buy them from a shop with a decent turnover of produce, then stash them in the fridge 'til I get round to using them.

### How to cook it

Pine nuts are a legendary component of pesto, and are equally at home in pasta dishes, too. Even more simply, lightly toasted they work a treat sprinkled on salads.

## Fresh pesto

Whilst you can get some decent tasting pesto by the jar, it's all too often a pale shade of what you can conjure from fresh. No doubt everyone has got their own way of doing this, but here's mine.

30 g (1 oz) pine nuts
60 g (2 oz) fresh basil leaves
1 garlic clove, chopped
Sea salt and black pepper
100 ml (3½ fl oz) extra virgin olive oil
   (plus a little extra to store)
30 g (1 oz) Parmesan, freshly grated

Start off by lightly toasting the pine nuts in a dry frying pan for a couple of minutes. Set aside to cool ■ You can do the next bit in a pestle and mortar, but for speed use a food processor. Blitz the pine nuts, basil and garlic until the basil and nuts look finely chopped. Season the mixture. With the processor running, gradually pour in about 75 ml (2¾ fl oz) of the olive oil, just until the oil is incorporated (I don't like my pesto to be too homogenous and over-processed, but you can play it by ear to suit your taste) ■ Transfer into a bowl and stir in the grated Parmesan. You can then stir in the remaining olive oil bit by bit until you get just the right consistency ■ Whatever pesto you have left can be stored in a covered jar in the fridge for a day or two, remembering to cover the top with a film of olive oil.

### Some variations

If you're an unwavering pesto purist you might want to look away now, but I'm not and I've tried – and thoroughly enjoyed – various adaptations on the pesto theme. These have involved swapping the pine nuts for almonds, cashew nuts or walnuts, the basil for rocket, or the Parmesan for Pecorino cheese. All proper lovely!

# Friends round

I reckon all those top chefs can teach us a thing or two about healthy eating. And that's the importance of fresh, local, seasonal produce. In short, quality ingredients produced with integrity. Okay, so there might be a bit too much salt, sugar or fat in some of their recipes, but I reckon if we all cooked more food from scratch using fresh, seasonal ingredients, we'd be a whole lot better off.

It also cuts to the chase of what this chapter is all about – letting lovely, fresh, seasonal ingredients do the talking and trying not to mess them up too much with a load of fancy stuff. I've also tried hard to moderate things like salt in these recipes, whilst making use of more 'good' fats in favour of too many 'bad' fats (although, I have to confess, sometimes only butter will do the trick!). All of that without making huge compromises in the taste department.

One way of achieving that is to make the best use of the array of amazing herbs and spices that most people tend not to use in their day-to-day cooking. They can do wonders when it comes to adding some jazz to a dish, the clincher being that they're also really good for you.

This chapter boils down to one thing. I want to change your mind about what 'healthy eating' is all about. For too long it's been synonymous with munching through a mountain of brown rice and tofu. Of course, there's nothing wrong with those particular foods, but if you're not careful it's going to be dull, bland and give you jaw-ache. And to be honest, all that righteous carrot crunching just isn't my thing. I'm more up for the serious business of actually enjoying healthy food. And I reckon you should be, too.

# Chicken

I'm not going to bang on too much about the animal welfare issues of intensive factory farming. Not because I don't think it's important, I totally do. It's just that others have been there and done it more eloquently than I ever could. That just leaves you to do the right thing.

### Why you should be eating it

Let's start with the obvious. Chicken provides a high-quality protein source needed for growth and repair of the body, and white meats such as chicken provide an alternative protein source to red meat. Whilst consumption of a lot of red meat and processed meat is linked to an increased risk of colorectal cancer, white meats such as chicken don't appear to be.

But, let's be aware that chicken may not be the super-healthy, high-protein, low fat food conventional nutritional wisdom touts it to be. Researchers have found that modern day chicken is much more fatty than a chicken would have been in the past, containing more calories and less protein. Not only has the amount of fat increased, but so has the actual type of fat, creating a less favourable balance of bad fats vs good fats. Hardly surprising if chickens are produced to gain weight rapidly on a cocktail of high-energy feed and minimal exercise.

Going for a free-range, traditionally reared bird is likely to go some way to providing healthier (and tastier) meat, and is a little closer to what nature intended.

### How to buy it

I said I wouldn't bang on about it. Free-range or organic whenever you can. Enough said.

### How to cook it

Roasting, baking, grilling, poaching, casseroles, soups, curries, stir-fries, yes. Reformed bits of chicken squashed together with a load of fillers into attractive little breadcrumb-coated shapes, no. And if you pay a bit more for a happy chicken, I'd urge you to be resourceful and make use of every last morsel of it, including making your own chicken stock from the carcass, which is never less than amazing.

## Chicken with 40 cloves of garlic

This has got to be at least 100 times better than a frozen chicken Kiev!

Serves 4

25 g (1 oz) unsalted butter
2 tbsp extra virgin olive oil
1 x 1.5 kg (3 lb) whole chicken, jointed
1 onion, thinly sliced
2 sticks of celery, thinly sliced
½ bottle of dry white wine, unchilled
40 garlic cloves, unpeeled
5 sprigs of thyme
3 bay leaves
1 sprig rosemary, 10 cm (4 in) long
Black pepper

Preheat the oven to 180ºC/350ºF/gas mark 4 ▣ Melt the butter in a deep-sided frying pan. Add the olive oil and fry the chicken pieces, two at a time, over a moderate heat to brown and crisp the skin. Remove and add to a large ovenproof casserole dish ▣ Add the onion and celery to the frying pan and fry until soft. Remove and add those to the casserole ▣ Add a splash of the white wine to the frying pan to deglaze, scraping up all the tasty brown bits to melt them into the wine. Once the pan has deglazed, add the rest of the wine and bring it up to boiling point, then pour the wine over the chicken and vegetables in the casserole ▣ Finally add the 40 cloves of unpeeled garlic, herbs and black pepper to the casserole. Cover and cook in the preheated oven for 1½ hours. Turn off the oven and leave to rest for 10 minutes with the door slightly ajar ▣ Great served with mashed potato and steamed veggies. As for the 40 cloves of garlic, simply squeeze them out of their papery husks and eat as many as you like.

# Venison

Venison comes big on flavour and it's healthy stuff. That's all my boxes ticked.

### Why you should be eating it

In terms of its health benefits, red meat is a bit of a double-edged sword. On the one hand, it packs an abundant source of nutrients such as protein, vitamin B12, and well-absorbed iron and zinc. On the other hand it tends to be high in saturated fat, which pushes up levels of 'bad' cholesterol. There's also substantial evidence that eating too much red meat is strongly linked with an increased risk of colon cancer.

The big bonus with venison is that, in contrast to more domesticated animals, it's a very lean meat, containing low levels of saturated fat. So effectively you are left with the good bits – the protein, the B-vitamins, the iron and zinc.

That's not to say that red meat, in whatever form, can be eaten with abandon, as the mechanisms relating to red meat consumption and cancer are quite complex. For example, the way we cook red meat may be an important factor, as high temperature cooking such as frying, grilling or barbecuing can lead to the formation of potentially cancer-causing substances known as heterocyclic amines and polycyclic aromatic hydrocarbons. It may even be the high levels of iron found in red meat that's problematic, as too much iron can lead to the production of damaging free radicals.

As with all of these things, it's about balance, and, all in all, I reckon venison has a lot going for it compared to other red meats.

### How to buy it

Quite a bit of the venison on sale is farmed rather than wild, but even then it would have most likely been grazing quite naturally. But if it's wild you're after, then your best bet will be a good butcher or game dealer.

### How to cook it

The thought of cooking game can be quite intimidating for the uninitiated, but it needn't be. You can eat venison as a steak, roast a joint, or use diced venison for hearty stews and casseroles. And home-made burgers, made with minced venison, are the business.

## Venison steaks

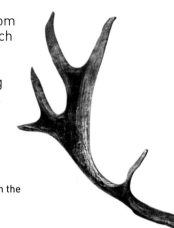

Venison steaks should come from either the haunch or the fillet and benefit from a little marinating for best results. And take care not to over-cook them.

### Serves 2

2 venison steaks from the haunch or fillet

FOR THE MARINADE
2 tbsp balsamic vinegar
2 garlic cloves, sliced
4 tbsp extra virgin olive oil
Zest of 1 unwaxed lemon
2 bay leaves

Mix all the ingredients for the marinade together in a non-metallic bowl. Immerse the steaks in the mixure, rubbing the marinade well into the grain of the meat. Cover and chill for at least an hour ▧ Heat a ridged griddle or frying pan until hot but not smoking. Place the steaks in the pan. They should immediately start to sizzle ▧ Cook to your liking, brushing on more of the marinade just before you turn them over ▧ Once cooked, place the steaks onto a warmed plate to rest for 5 minutes covered with foil, then serve.

# Lamb

Whilst red meat has fallen out of favour it can supply a lot of useful nutrients. Just be sure to eat it sparingly.

## Why you should be eating it

Straight down to business. Lamb is packed with protein, vitamin B12 and the minerals zinc and iron. Let's start with zinc, needed for everything from immunity, to fertility, to growth. Not only does lamb provide a good bit of zinc, it appears that the presence of animal protein at a meal actually increases its absorption.

Lamb is a plentiful source of iron. Not just any old iron, but a type of iron called 'haem' iron, which is absorbed a whole lot more efficiently than 'non-haem' iron found in plant foods. Whilst many people get plenty of iron (it is present in all manner of plant-based foods after all, not just meat), some groups appear to be at greater risk of iron deficiency, a good example being younger women. And ultimately, the consequence of not getting enough iron is anaemia.

Now, there's a big caveat here. Lamb is also high in saturated fat, and eating a lot of red meat is likely to increase the risk of heart disease and certain types of cancer, notably of the colon. Time for the old cliché. You guessed it – all things in moderation.

## How to buy it

Lamb farming is much less intensive than, say, poultry farming, and that's undoubtedly a good thing. If your pockets are deep enough, you might want to pay that bit extra for organic lamb, which is always a good bet.

## How to cook it

Grilling, roasting, slow-cooking, stews, casseroles, home-made kebabs or a good old shepherd's pie spring to mind. In terms of the healthiest way to cook lamb, slower cooking at lower temperatures (think stews and casseroles) is better than high temperature cooking which leads to charred or burnt meat. The latter leads to the formation of harmful chemicals that have been associated with increased cancer risk.

## Slow-cooked lamb tagine

This is definitely not fast food, but well worth the wait, and the vast array of phytochemicals found in all those spices and herbs bump up the health credentials big-time.

Serves 4

1 tbsp olive oil
450 g (1 lb) diced lamb
Sea salt and black pepper
1 large onion, finely chopped
1 tsp cinnamon
1 tsp ginger
1 tsp paprika
¼ tsp cayenne pepper
¼ tsp crushed saffron threads
350 ml (12 fl oz) vegetable stock
1 x 400 g (14 oz) tin chopped tomatoes
½ tbsp clear honey
16 dates, pitted and quartered
1 x 400 g (14 oz) tin chickpeas, drained and rinsed
1 handful fresh coriander (cilantro), roughly chopped

Heat the olive oil in a large, deep saucepan. Add the lamb, season with a little sea salt and black pepper and cook until the lamb is browned. Remove the lamb and set aside ■ Add the onion to the saucepan and sauté for roughly 5 minutes until translucent and tender. Mix in the cinnamon, ginger, paprika, cayenne pepper and saffron. If the mixture is getting too dry, add a splash of water ■ Return the lamb to the pan and combine well with the spice mixture. Add the vegetable stock, tomatoes, honey, dates and chickpeas. Bring to the boil ■ Cover and gently simmer on a low heat for 1½–2 hours, stirring occasionally, until the lamb is really tender. If it starts to dry out, just add a splash more water or stock ■ Stir in the coriander and serve ■ Couscous makes the ideal accompaniment, or less conventionally, I love this with a big, fat baked sweet potato.

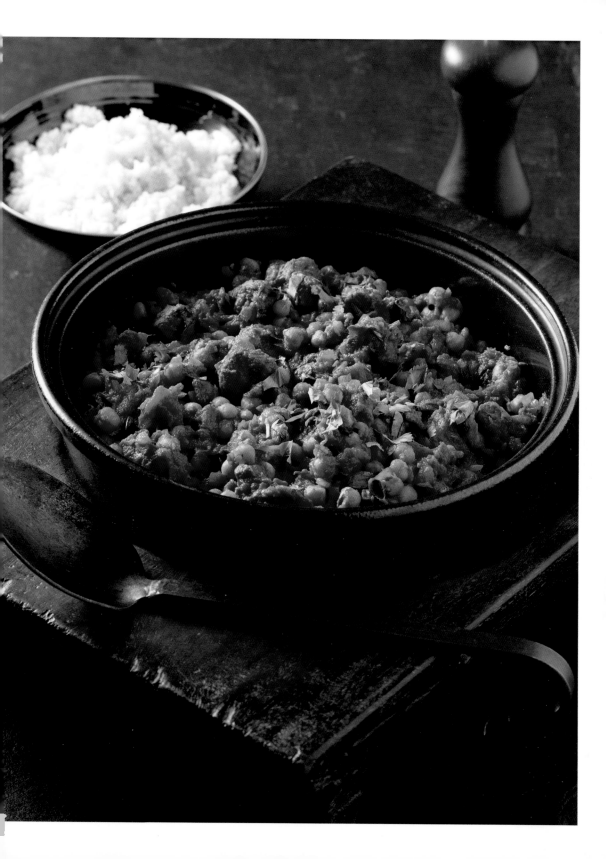

# Salmon

I look upon salmon as being the acceptable face of oily fish – the one oily fish that you can generally get people to eat even if they won't go near mackerel or sardines.

## Why you should be eating it

Here I'll be giving a lowdown on the anti-inflammatory properties of oily fish. But if you want to know more about its nutrient content, then take a trip to anchovies on page 48, for its heart health credentials, hit mackerel on page 56, and if you're hungry for more, see sardines on page 58 for the lowdown on its reputation as brain food.

Excessive inflammation contributes to many common health problems. The good news is that the omega-3 fats found in oily fish can help reduce inflammatory reactions in the body. For example, in rheumatoid arthritis evidence indicates that omega-3 fish oils may offer some symptomatic relief to sufferers. There's also evidence to suggest benefits in other conditions such as inflammatory bowel disease or asthma, although the evidence isn't very strong and more research needs to be done to gain a better understanding.

But the bottom line is that typical Western diets lean towards too much omega-6 fats relative to omega-3 fats, and this imbalance may be exacerbating inflammatory health problems. The anti-inflammatory actions of omega-3 fats, low in most modern diets, acts as a useful counterbalance.

## How to buy it

Most salmon is intensively farmed, not dissimilar to factory farmed poultry. I know it hits your pocket harder, but I'd encourage either organic salmon (still farmed, but to higher standards) or better still the wild stuff (making sure it's from sustainable fisheries – look out for Marine Stewardship Council certification).

## How to cook it

Whether you bake it, grill it, pan-fry it, poach it, steam it, or barbecue it, the secret to great tasting salmon is not to overcook it.

## Grilled wild salmon with caper sauce

When it comes to fish, buy it fresh, cook it fresh, and don't mess around with it too much. In short, keep it simple and let the quality of the ingredients do the talking.

### Serves 4

4 good size wild salmon fillets
    (around 150 g/5 oz each)
20 g (¾ oz) butter, melted
Sea salt and black pepper

FOR THE CAPER SAUCE
4 tbsp natural yoghurt
40 g (1½ oz) capers, finely chopped
25 g (1 oz) fresh chives, finely chopped

Brush the salmon with the melted butter, season to taste, and place under a hot grill. Cook for approximately 4–5 minutes on the flesh side and 2 minutes on the skin side ■ That just gives you time to quickly throw together the caper sauce. Simply combine all the ingredients and mix well ■ When the salmon is cooked, serve immediately accompanied by a generous spoonful or two of the caper sauce on the side ■ Great served with new potatoes and green beans.

### EATING OILY FISH

Oily fish have the potential to accumulate various pollutants such as polychlorinated biphenyls (PCBs) and dioxins. To ensure the benefits of eating oily fish, of which there are many, outweigh potential risks, it is recommended that women who are pregnant or breastfeeding, or girls and women who may become pregnant at some point in their lives, should avoid eating more than two portions of oily fish per week. For everyone else, eating up to four portions of oily fish per week is unlikely to pose a problem.

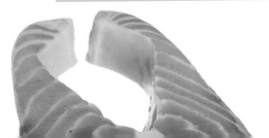

# Cod

I'm no expert on the sustainability of fish, but I do try to do my bit. There are big concerns that cod stocks are dwindling. But it's now possible to get sustainable cod – so do your bit, too, and look out for the Marine Stewardship Council logo before you buy.

### Why you should be eating it

Cod offers a cracking source of high-quality protein. Of course, the real bonus here is that compared with meat, levels of saturated fat are much lower. It also contributes valuable iodine to the diet. This trace element is important for making thyroid hormones, which play a hugely important role in maintaining a healthy metabolic rate. And if you don't have enough of these hormones you'll be prone to a plethora of symptoms such as lethargy, weight gain, poor concentration, dry skin and low mood, to name but a few.

Cod also provides abundant B-vitamins, notably B12. This is quite an odd-one-out, insofar as it's almost exclusively found in animal foods, rather than plant foods. Amongst its many functions it works in collaboration with folic acid and vitamin B6 to control levels of homocysteine in the bloodstream, elevations of which are linked with heart disease risk.

Last but by no means least, cod provides a top notch source of selenium, important for immune function, thyroid function, fertility and reproductive health, our antioxidant defences, and probably cancer prevention, too. And there's a big debate in some countries as to whether we're getting enough to meet our needs for optimal health.

### How to buy it

If in doubt about the sustainability of your cod, you could happily give pollack a go instead.

### How to cook it

Cod is really versatile. Grill, bake, poach or pan-fry it, remembering not to overcook it.

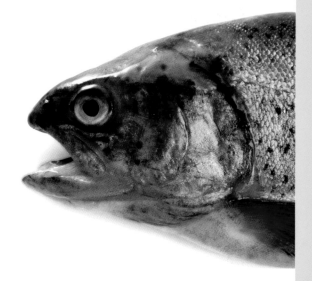

## Louise's baked cod in red pepper sauce

My other half, Louise, reckons she can't cook. One day she randomly 'threw together' this little number. Genius! What's she on about?

Serves 4

600 g (1½ lb) skinless cod fillet
2 red (bell) peppers, deseeded and roughly chopped
1 medium red onion, roughly chopped
1 red chilli, deseeded and roughly chopped
2 garlic cloves, crushed
2 tbsp extra virgin olive oil
Sea salt and black pepper
60 ml (2 fl oz) water

Cut the cod into four equal pieces and place in a large baking dish ■ Blitz all the other ingredients in a blender until smooth. Pour evenly over the fish ■ Cook uncovered at 190°C/375°F/gas mark 5 for 35 minutes, making sure the fish is thoroughly cooked through ■ Serve with new potatoes and a fresh green salad.

# Duck

Given the choice of wild game or intensively factory farmed meat, I'd go with wild every time. And if there was only factory farmed meat on offer, I'd go vegetarian.

## Why you should be eating it

If you've never sampled a wild quacker then give it a go. It's a whole lot different to the more fatty domesticated duck that you might be accustomed to. After all, these are birds that actually swim and fly around as part of their day job (the true meaning of free range). And the meat is much leaner as a result.

That stacks up to all the nutritional benefits of eating meat, with less of the pitfalls. With wild duck you'll be getting a plentiful supply of high-quality protein, the minerals iron and selenium, along with a good range of B-vitamins, notably B12. All without the higher levels of fat that you might find in more domestically reared birds.

## How to buy it

Wild duck refers mainly to either mallard or teal. That means a trip to your local game dealer. And there are loads of good independent butchers around that sell game. Depending on its size (and your appetite!), one mallard should provide plenty of meat for two. Or you can just buy mallard breasts instead.

## How to cook it

Wild duck makes for a lovely alternative to roast chicken, beef or lamb.

# Roasted mallard with orange and fennel

A wild mallard makes for a perfect dinner for two.

### Serves 2

25 g (1 oz) unsalted butter
1 fennel bulb, thinly sliced
4 garlic cloves, peeled and lightly crushed
Small bunch of fresh thyme
2 bay leaves
1 wild mallard, approx 1 kg (2 lb) in weight
1 unwaxed orange
Black pepper
200 ml (7 fl oz) red wine
25 g (1 oz) unsalted butter, chilled and diced

Preheat the oven to 200°C/400°F/gas mark 6. Melt the butter in a roasting tin and fry the sliced fennel, garlic, thyme and bay leaves until the edges of the fennel just start turning golden brown ■ Wash the duck inside and out, pat dry with kitchen paper. Cut the orange in half. Take one half, slice it thinly and use the slices to cover the breast of the bird ■ Place the duck on top of the sautéed fennel. Zest the other half of the orange, reserve and then juice. Pour over the orange juice and red wine, season with black pepper and roast until cooked, roughly 40–45 minutes. Leave it to rest, breast turned down and covered in foil in a warm spot ■ Meanwhile, take the roasting tin with the fennel and red wine and bring to the boil to reduce slightly. Start whisking in the chilled diced butter, a piece at a time to give the sauce a gloss. Once the butter has been added, stir in the reserved orange zest and simmer for 2 minutes. Remove the bay leaf and thyme ■ Carve the duck and serve with the fennel on the side and the hot sauce poured over the top.

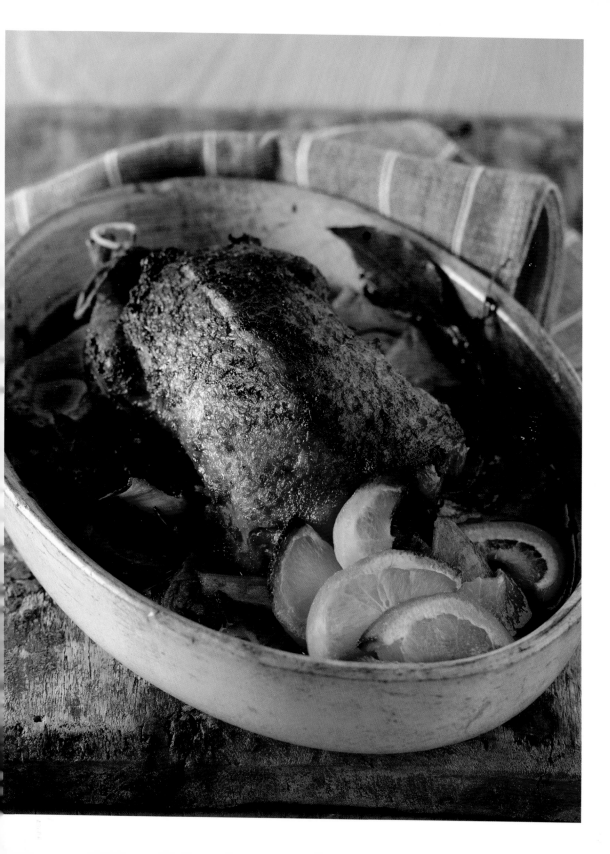

# The spice rack

I'm a big fan of using a few well-chosen herbs and spices in my cooking, but thanks to our over-reliance on ready-made convenience food it's something that most people don't do enough of. Salt and pepper is about as adventurous as most of us get, and that's a shame as culinary herbs and spices are packed full of beneficial plant compounds, a bit like those you'd find in fruits and vegetables. That might go some way to explaining why many of them are highly prized for their medicinal and curative properties in traditional folk medicine, and good-old science is now helping us to better understand how and why some of these active ingredients may benefit health.

There are loads of amazing herbs and spices out there. Here are just a few that I wouldn't be without in the kitchen.

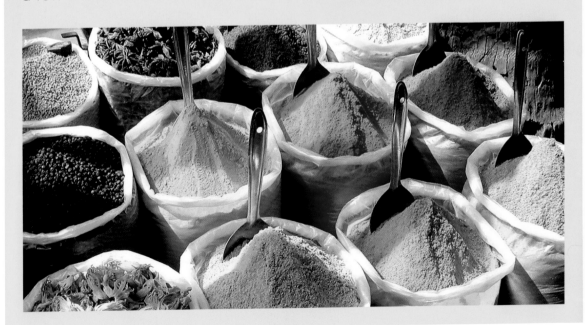

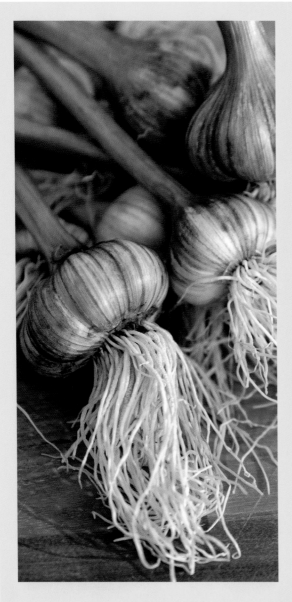

such as rheumatoid arthritis and inflammatory bowel disease, amongst others.

It may just turn out to be brain food, too, with mounting experimental evidence that curcumin may help protect against Alzheimer's disease by reducing inflammation and the build-up of the characteristic plaque seen in the brain of Alzheimer's disease sufferers. Indeed, regular consumption of this spice may go some way to explaining the lower prevalence of this disease in India.

But we shouldn't get too carried away. The active stuff in turmeric, the curcumin, has poor bio-availability, which means it's not absorbed very well when we consume it and what little we do absorb is got rid of pretty quick. At the moment most of the research is fancy stuff done in a lab, or on animals and not real life humans, so there's still loads to find out about how it might be used to improve our health. But all said and done, not a bad reason (like you ever needed one) to get busy making a curry.

## Garlic

Most people either love or loathe garlic. It's renowned for its cardio-protective credentials, with some evidence to suggest that regular consumption may hold benefits for preventing or slowing cardiovascular disease. Such benefits include lowering elevated cholesterol levels, reducing the stickiness of the blood, and protection against atherosclerosis and the build-up of plaque on the inside of artery walls. That said, the evidence is pretty shaky and far from conclusive, so I wouldn't pin too much hope on the idea that adding a bit of garlic to your diet will make a massive difference.

There's also been more than a sniff of interest in the potential anti-cancer properties of garlic. Whilst it's really difficult to study these things accurately in humans, regularly incorporating garlic into the diet appears to be associated with protection against certain types of cancer such as stomach cancer, and most notably, colorectal cancer.

## Turmeric

Turmeric is the yellow-orange spice of curry fame. Its active constituent, curcumin, has been hot stuff amongst researchers with an interest in its possible health benefits. That's because curcumin has been shown to possess antioxidant, anti-inflammatory and even anti-cancer properties, and this has led to interest in its potential application in numerous ailments

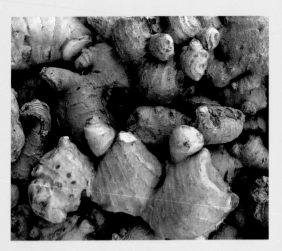

## Ginger

Ginger has traditionally been revered for both its culinary and medicinal properties. Amongst its health benefits, ginger has a reputation for alleviating nausea, along with being a folk remedy for easing digestive problems. It's also made a name for itself as a natural anti-inflammatory, and has a history of traditional use for ailments such as aches, pains and arthritis.

Modern day scientific research is beginning to catch up with what ancient folk medicine has known for ages. As one might expect from such a spicy little number, numerous bio-active compounds have been identified in ginger, such as the pungent gingerols and shogaols. That ginger has been shown to possess significant antioxidant and anti-inflammatory properties may go some way to explaining its long-standing reputation as a restorative folk remedy.

## Chilli and cayenne pepper

Whilst you're not likely to catch me eating a vindaloo (I prefer my taste buds intact), I am partial to a bit of zing in my food by way of a dash of chilli. Used fittingly, a little bit of chilli can make a world of difference to a dish. What makes chilli hot property is its active constituent

capsaicin. Most of the attention for this chilli compound has focused on its topical use in analgesic ointments for certain types of nerve pain where it's thought to work by helping to block pain signals from the body to the brain.

Alongside interest in its anti-inflammatory and analgesic properties, there is some evidence that regular ingestion of chilli, and its active constituent capsaicin, may play a role in assisting weight loss through helping the body burn more energy. That said, I reckon there's probably easier and more effective ways of shedding a few pounds.

Whilst cayenne pepper has traditionally been regarded as a digestive stimulant, don't go overboard with the hot stuff as too much might potentially act as an irritant in the stomach, with some evidence, albeit pretty inconclusive and inconsistent, that high intakes might be associated with an increased risk of stomach cancer.

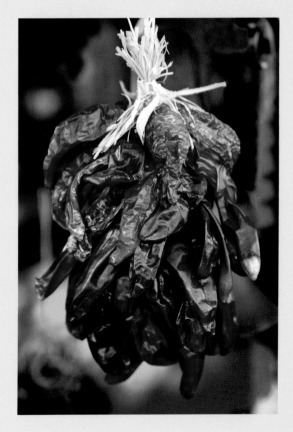

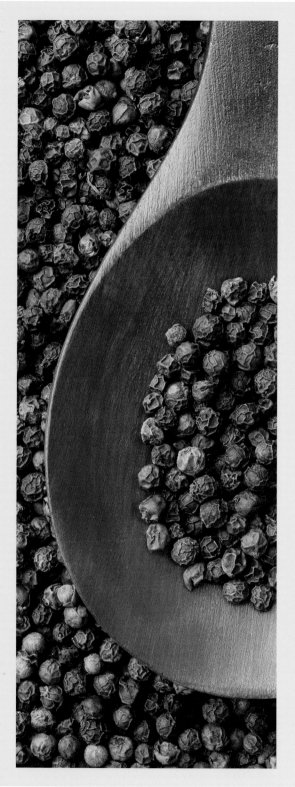

## Black pepper

Whilst I'm a big fan of making good use of a whole range of culinary spices in cooking, black pepper is a trusty household name that most folk will be well familiar with. Exotic it might not be, but it's a spice that grabs the attention for reasons other than flavour alone.

The principle active constituent of black pepper is a pungent alkaloid called piperine. Researchers who have been investigating this compound have uncovered effects as diverse as stimulating digestion and improving absorption, antioxidant properties, anti-depressant like effects, and a whole lot more besides.

That's not to say that a sprinkling of the freshly ground stuff at the dinner table will have all those benefits. Lab experiments using isolated extracts are very different to real life dietary intakes after all. But it's interesting to think that a humdrum spice like black pepper contains such intriguing components.

## Garam masala

For the uninitiated, garam masala is a blend of warming spices with diverse uses in Indian cooking. Whilst there's no definitive recipe for exactly what goes into garam masala (it varies according to region), it might contain some of the spices I've been banging on about here, such as black peppercorns, in combination with other antioxidant and phytochemical-rich spices such as cumin seeds, coriander seeds, cinnamon or cloves, and more besides.

In a way, a bit like with fruit and veggies, having a good variety of culinary spices means that you get to take on board a complex and synergistic mix of beneficial plant compounds. I reckon that Hippocrates was definitely on to something all those years back when he piped up with that 'Let food be thy medicine' catchphrase. And that's probably never been more relevant than it is today.

# Mozzarella

Whilst I won't pretend cheese is super-healthy, mozzarella is a calcium-packed fast food.

## Why you should be eating it

What do you want first, the good news or the bad news? I'll stick with tradition and do the bad news first. Mozzarella, like many cheeses, is fairly high in saturated fat. That's the sort of fat that pushes up cholesterol levels and in excess can contribute to heart disease.

But I don't think it's really about hailing one food as good, and condemning another as bad. It's about looking at whole diets. And mozzarella does have some good stuff to offer. For starters, it's packed full of high-quality protein, needed for growth and repair of the body.

And like dairy products in general, it contains loads of calcium. We already know that getting enough of this mineral is really important for developing and maintaining strong bones. But calcium has other strings to its bow, with evidence accumulating to show that a calcium-rich diet may have a role to play in reducing body weight and body fat, and thus protecting against obesity. Saying that, common sense would suggest low fat dairy products are a better bet than their full fat counterparts when it comes to matters of the waistline.

## How to buy it

Traditionally, mozzarella is made from water buffalo milk, and that will most likely be the artisan's choice every time. But nowadays it's often made from cow's milk, too.

## How to cook it

Accompanied by tomatoes, basil and olive oil, mozzarella can be turned into a lip-smacker of a starter or salad. When it comes to cooking, it's commonly used as a pizza topping, in pasta dishes, but also a variety of other meat and vegetable recipes, too.

# Smoked haddock fishcakes with mozzarella

If you're a bit unsure about whether or not you like fish, I reckon you should give this a whirl.

### Serves 2

400 g (14 oz) floury potatoes (e.g. Desiree, King Edward, Maris Piper), peeled and chopped
225 g (8 oz) smoked haddock
300 ml (½ pt) semi-skimmed (2% milkfat) milk
Black pepper
25 g (1 oz) unsalted butter
5 spring onions (scallions), thickly sliced
2 tbsp capers, roughly chopped
Small handful of fresh basil, torn
115 g (4 oz) bag of fresh mozzarella, diced
Small pinch of salt
1 free range egg, lightly beaten
70 g (3 oz) wholemeal (whole-wheat) breadcrumbs (2 slices of bread)
1 tsp extra virgin olive oil
Lemon wedges, to serve

Add the potatoes to a large pan, cover with water, bring to the boil and simmer until tender ■ Put the haddock into a frying pan (this needs to be large enough to hold the fish in one layer), pour the milk over and season with black pepper. Bring to a gentle simmer and poach. The fish is cooked once you can separate the white flakes easily with the tip of a knife. Remove the fish from the frying pan, reserving the milk, and peel the skin away. Flake the fish into small pieces in a bowl, removing any bones as you go ■ The potatoes should be done now. Mash them roughly with the butter and a little of the reserved milk. Keep the mash rough, not smooth or else the fishcakes will fall apart ■ Mix the potatoes with the fish, spring onions, capers, basil, mozzarella and season. Make four cakes about 2 cm (¾ in) thick ■ You're now ready to cook the fishcakes. Place the lightly beaten egg into a bowl and the breadcrumbs onto a plate. Dip each fishcake into the egg first and then into the crumbs, making sure they're well coated all over ■ Heat the olive oil in a non stick frying pan. Fry the fishcakes for 10 minutes on each side until golden brown and well heated through ■ Serve straight away with the lemon wedges on the side.

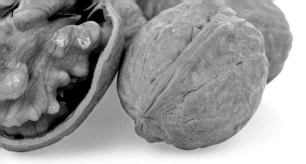

# Walnuts

Walnuts. A calorie counters worst nightmare, right? Seeing foods simply in terms of how many calories they contain is a bit of a mistake. Do that and you may just miss the bigger picture.

### Why you should be eating it

Nuts are a high fat food. No argument there. But we're talking here almost entirely about 'good' fats, of the polyunsaturated and monounsaturated kind. And as it goes, walnuts are one of the relatively few plant foods to contain meaningful amounts of the much sought after omega-3 fats. This favourable balance of beneficial fats accounts in part for the cardio-protective reputation of walnuts.

But the health benefits of walnuts are not just down to all those good fats. Whilst we tend to associate antioxidants with eating fruit and veg, walnuts are a mighty source of these protective compounds, and right up there as one of the highest dietary sources. More reason, if ever you needed it, to include more plant foods, not just fruit and veg, in the diet.

Of course, there's a whole lot more to walnuts, also packing a stash of vitamins, minerals, fibre, phytochemicals and cholesterol-lowering phytosterols.

### How to buy it

Remember that all those good fats are prone to going rancid, so I recommend storing shelled walnuts in an airtight container in the fridge to maintain maximum freshness.

### How to cook it

Walnuts are great just as they are to banish hunger pangs, as well as working a treat chopped and sprinkled on to muesli, porridge, yoghurt, salads or grain-based dishes.

## Vegetable nut crumble

This savoury take on crumble is proof that there's more to veggie food than beans and lentils.

**Serves 4**

FOR THE VEGETABLE FILLING
2 tbsp extra virgin olive oil
1 large onion, roughly chopped
450 g (1 lb) mixed root vegetables (such as parsnips, carrots, turnips and swede), peeled and chopped
25 g (1 oz) wholemeal plain (whole-wheat all-purpose) flour
1 x 400 g (14 oz) tin of chopped tomatoes
200 ml (7 fl oz) semi-skimmed (2% milkfat) milk
1 tsp vegetable stock powder
1 tsp dried thyme
2 bay leaves
Black pepper
2 tbsp finely chopped fresh parsley

FOR THE CRUMBLE
100 g (4 oz) unsalted butter, chilled and cut into cubes
175 g (6 oz) wholemeal plain (whole-wheat all-purpose) flour
50 g (2 oz) Parmesan, grated
75 g (3 oz) mixed nuts and seeds (such as walnuts, hazelnuts, sesame seeds and sunflower seeds), chopped

Heat the oil in a large pan and gently soften the chopped onion. Add the vegetables, cover and cook over a gentle heat for 15 minutes, stirring occasionally. Stir in the flour and cook again for 1 minute, stirring constantly. Add the tomatoes, milk, stock powder, thyme, bay leaves and pepper. Bring to the boil, stirring all the time as the sauce thickens. Reduce the heat, cover and cook until the vegetables are tender, approximately 20 minutes. When ready, stir in the chopped parsley ■ Preheat the oven to 190ºC/375ºF/gas mark 5 ■ While the filling is simmering, make the crumble topping. Rub the butter into the flour. It's best to use your fingers but you can whizz it in a blender. Stir in the grated Parmesan and mixed chopped nuts and seeds ■ Once the vegetables are tender and the crumble mix ready, pour the vegetables and their sauce into an ovenproof dish roughly 23 cm (9 in) in diameter. Spoon the crumble mix lightly over the vegetables – don't press it down. Place in the oven and cook for 30 minutes.

# Chickpeas

We tend to be a bit meat obsessed and in so being overlook other sources of protein from the plant world, such as pulses. Nutritional nuggets like chickpeas could make a welcome addition to the typical westernized diet.

### Why you should be eating it

Let's kick off with the obvious one. Fibre. The stuff most of us eating Western diets don't really get enough of, and chickpeas contain oodles of it.

There are some pretty obvious benefits of fibre in terms of digestive health. No prizes for guessing what they are. But perhaps less well known are some of fibre's other attributes, with a good bit of evidence showing that higher intakes are associated with a lower risk of heart disease. One of the ways this is achieved is through a cholesterol-lowering effect of fibre, notably a specific type called soluble-fibre. And pulses such as chickpeas are noteworthy sources of the soluble type, helping to explain their reputation as a handy food when it comes to keeping levels of 'bad' LDL-cholesterol in check.

Let's not forget that chickpeas are also a great source of vegetarian protein, B-vitamins such as folate, and minerals, including iron. And just to testify to the funky array of compounds we find in plant foods, pulses such as chickpeas are packed with a whole load of other stuff such as resistant starch, phytosterols and isoflavones, all of which may have the potential to influence our health for the better.

### How to buy it

The big debate: dried vs canned. All that soaking and boiling is quite a palaver, but I reckon they do taste better that way. But mostly, I don't have time to be that much of a purist and just opt for the pre-cooked canned variety avoiding the ones with added sugar or salt.

### How to cook it

Chickpeas are a big part of Middle Eastern and Indian dishes. Think no further than hummus, falafels and curries. But they're also great added to stews, casseroles, soups, even salads.

## Chickpea and spinach curry (Chana Sag)

Total proof that curry can be right up there as a health food.

### Serves 4

1 tbsp groundnut oil
1 onion, thinly sliced
2 garlic cloves, finely chopped
1 x 400 g (14 oz) tin of tomatoes, whizzed in a blender
1 green chilli, deseeded and finely chopped
5 cm (2 in) piece of fresh ginger, peeled and grated
1 tsp turmeric
1 tsp garam masala
¼ tsp sea salt
Good handful of fresh coriander (cilantro), chopped
Dash of lemon juice
2 x 400 g (14 oz) tins chickpeas, drained and rinsed
150 g (5 oz) spinach, washed and shredded
4 spring onions (scallions), finely chopped

Heat the groundnut oil over a moderate heat and fry the onion and garlic until golden brown ■ Turn down the heat and add the tomatoes, chilli, ginger, turmeric, garam masala, salt, coriander and lemon juice. Stir well and add a splash of water. Keep stirring for a few minutes and then add the chickpeas. Add enough water to cover and bring to the boil ■ Simmer for 15 minutes, then add the spinach and simmer for another 5 minutes. If the sauce looks too watery, simmer for a further 5 minutes or so ■ Serve once the spinach is cooked topped with the chopped spring onions. Brown basmati rice or Bombay potatoes would make a perfect accompaniment.

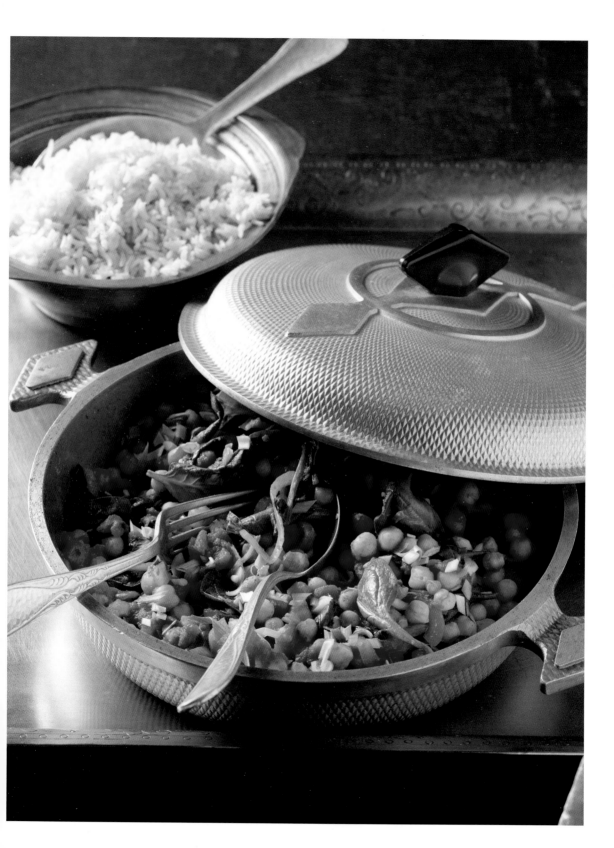

# Spelt

Spelt is an ancient type of wheat that's made a name for itself in recent years. Some people who don't get on all that well with wheat report that they are able to better tolerate spelt, but just for the record, it is a type of wheat and it does contain gluten.

## Why you should be eating it

There's every reason to think that consuming spelt will carry the same health benefits as other wholegrains. These are not inconsiderable, with evidence indicating an association between consumption of wholegrains and a reduced risk of such notable chronic health problems as heart disease, some cancers, diabetes and obesity. The same, however, can't be said for eating grains in their 'white' refined state.

Taking grains such as spelt in the wholegrain form means they're a whole lot more nutritious. And that doesn't just mean the standard vitamins and minerals, which are found aplenty in spelt, either. Wholegrain cereals, just like other plant foods, are jam-packed with other beneficial phytochemicals, antioxidants and of course, stacks of fibre.

## How to buy it

Spelt has catapulted from health food curiosity to mainstream fame, with widely available spelt versions of standard wheat classics to be found lining the shelves of many a shop and supermarket.

## How to cook it

Anything that you would normally do with wholemeal flour, you can do with spelt flour. It makes for a lovely rustic loaf, is great for pizza bases and home baking generally.

## Spelt bread pizza with goat's cheese, black olives and wilted rocket

With the right ingredients, I reckon pizza can be regarded as a health food, not a junk food. And if you want to totally cheat, you can buy pre-made spelt pizza bases.

Serves 2

FOR THE BASE
8 g (¼ oz) fresh yeast
1 tsp honey
200 ml (7 fl oz) warm water
250 g (9 oz) stoneground spelt flour
½ tsp sea salt
1 tbsp extra virgin olive oil

FOR THE TOMATO SAUCE
1 tbsp extra virgin olive oil
1 onion, finely chopped
1 garlic clove, crushed
350 g (12 oz) tomato passata (tomato sauce)
1 tbsp tomato purée (tomato paste)
½ tsp dried oregano
½ tsp dried basil
1 tsp brown sugar
Sea salt and black pepper

FOR THE TOPPING
200 g (7 oz) soft goat's cheese
Handful of black olives, pitted and halved
2 large handfuls rocket (arugula)
Extra virgin olive oil, for drizzling

Blend the yeast with the honey and half the water before mixing with the flour in a large bowl. Dissolve the salt in the remaining water before adding to the flour mixture. Add the olive oil and stir with a wooden spoon for 10–15 minutes. Allow the dough to rise in a warm place for 20-25 mins ■ Lightly grease a baking tray (either one really big one, or two smaller ones) and roll the dough in to two thin circular bases 20 cm (8-9 in) across. If the dough is too sticky knead in a little extra flour. Bake in a preheated oven (180°C/350°F/gas mark 5) for 15 minutes ■ Meanwhile, make the sauce. Heat the olive oil and gently fry the onions and garlic until soft and translucent. Add the tomato passata, tomato purée, dried herbs and brown sugar and season to taste. Simmer for around 10 mins ■ Add generous amounts of the tomato sauce to the pizza bases. Crumble the goat's cheese over the pizzas and arrange the black olives. Return the pizza to the oven and bake for 8 minutes ■ Remove the pizzas and scatter a handful of rocket leaves over each one. Return to the oven for a few seconds and remove just as the rocket begins to wilt ■ Drizzle with olive oil, season with black pepper and serve.

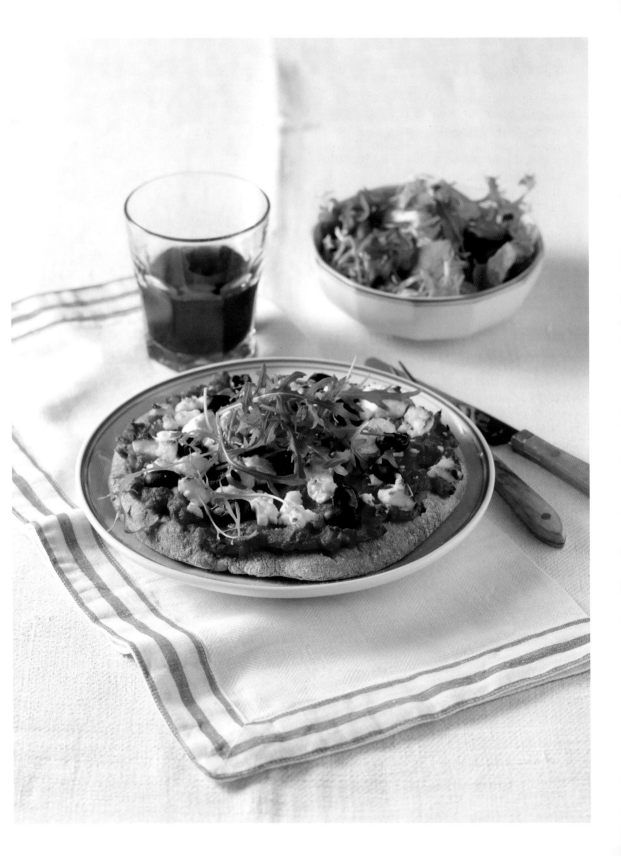

# Broccoli

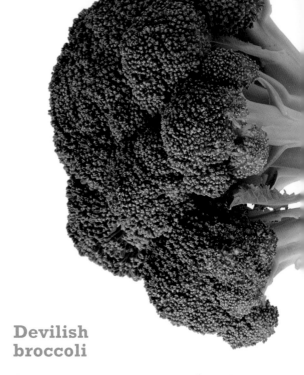

Broccoli must be good for you. Tell you why, I've heard one of the stallholders at my local market hailing its anti-cancer properties to his would-be punters. And I'll bet that helped shift a few more kilos that day.

### Why you should be eating it

Broccoli appears to contain compounds that help the body deal with potential cancer-causing substances. Broccoli hails from the cruciferous family of vegetables, distinguished for being uniquely rich in beneficial plant compounds called glucosinolates. When we eat broccoli, these get converted into the more active isothiocyanates, such as sulforaphane, which are thought to exert cancer-protective effects in the body, helping to explain the association between regular consumption of cruciferous veggies and a lowered risk of common cancers.

Broccoli's other virtues include good levels of a number of other nutrients, namely a decent bit of dietary fibre, antioxidant vitamin C, bone-friendly vitamin K, homocysteine-lowering folate, along with eye protective carotenoids lutein and zeaxanthin.

### How to buy it

The fresher the better. And if it's the lovely lush local, seasonal stuff plucked straight out the field you're after, then farm shops and farmers markets are always a good bet.

### How to cook it

Green veg doesn't always go down well with people, but a bit of creativity can go a long way. So I'm up for adding some jazz to proceedings in the form of fresh herbs, garlic, ginger or other spices. And please, I beg you, try to avoid boiling broccoli to a miserable mush.

## Devilish broccoli

Broccoli isn't exactly the rock 'n' roll of the food world. Time to big-up its reputation with some bold flavours. This recipe poses the risk of broccoli becoming the nicest tasting thing on your plate.

### Serves 4

1 large head of broccoli, cut into florets and thickly sliced
2 tbsp extra virgin olive oil
¼ tsp dried chilli flakes
½ tsp cumin seeds
½ tsp crushed coriander seeds
1 large onion, halved and finely sliced
1 fresh red chilli, deseeded and finely chopped
A pinch of sea salt
A handful of fresh coriander (cilantro), chopped

Steam the broccoli florets for approximately 3 minutes. Take care not to over-cook them – they should still be firm and crunchy ■ Meanwhile heat the olive oil in a large frying pan and add the dried chilli flakes, cumin and coriander seeds and gently fry for about 30 seconds ■ Add the sliced onion and gently fry until the onion turns translucent. Add the broccoli, fresh chilli and sea salt and continue to cook for a further 5 minutes ■ Stir-in the coriander and serve immediately.

# Carrots

With their help-you-see-in-the-dark
reputation, it was a dead cert that carrots
would pop up somewhere along the way.

## Why you should be eating it

Carrots are prized for their exceptionally high
content of carotenoids, notably beta carotene,
responsible for the vegetables' characteristic bright
orange hue. Beta carotene acts as an antioxidant in
its own right, but can also be converted in the body
into vitamin A, an important vitamin for maintaining
healthy skin not only on the outside, but also the
mucus linings on the inside, such as those of the
airways and the digestive system. Vitamin A also
helps to strengthen the immune system, whilst a
lack of it leads to poor vision in dim light, hence the
carrot's see-in-the-dark infamy.

But beta carotene has also been the subject of
intense research in its own right. A high intake of
beta carotene-rich foods (and we're talking fruits
and veggies here, not in pill form) is associated with
a reduced risk of some of the major killers in the
Western world, namely heart disease and cancer.

## How to buy it

I reckon carrots are one of the vegetables where
organic definitely taste better. If I was to do the
equivalent of the Pepsi taste challenge with
carrots, I reckon I'd have no problem identifying
the organic one. But even they're still no match
for the ones my mum grows in her back garden,
which are in a different class!

## How to cook it

Whilst you can boil or steam carrots, I reckon they
can be a bit bland that way (my mum's carrots
being the exception). So I prefer roasting them or
using them for hearty soups and casseroles. Finely
grated, they also add great texture and colour to
just about any salad.

## Honey-roasted carrots

If you can get hold of long, thin carrots
for this, perfect, just use them whole.
If not, just use chunky carrots cut in
half lengthways.

Serves 4

600 g (1½ lb) carrots
1 tbsp clear honey
1 tbsp olive oil
1 tsp caraway seeds
Sea salt and black pepper

Wash or peel the carrots and cut lengthways as
necessary. Steam them until just tender, roughly
10–15 minutes. Don't overcook them, they should
retain a bit of bite ■ Transfer to a roasting tin and
coat really well with the honey, olive oil, caraway
seeds and seasoning ■ Roast in a preheated oven
at 200°C/400°F/gas mark 6 for about 20 minutes
until the carrots begin to look golden.

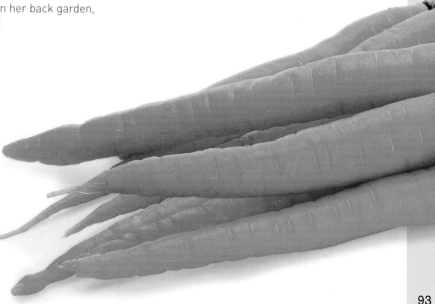

# Kale

When you see a vegetable this green and leafy, it can only mean one thing – it's got to be ridiculously good for you.

## Why you should be eating it

It's difficult to know where to begin, as the nutritional content of kale reads a bit like the label of a pot of multivitamin pills. In fact, it'd probably be easier to tell you what kale hasn't got in it. Judging by its deep green colour, you'd think kale would be full of antioxidants. And you'd be spot on, with kale muscling in with the big timers, such as blueberries.

Dark green leafy veg like kale are also a cracking source of carotenoids. These include antioxidant beta carotene, but also stomping amounts of eye-friendly lutein and zeaxanthin.

When we think of bone-building foods, milk and dairy products spring to mind. But kale comes up trumps not only with a respectable bit of calcium, but bags full of vitamin K, which also has a role to play in promoting strong and healthy bones.

Kale is a cruciferous vegetable hailing from the same family of vegetables as cabbage, broccoli, Brussels sprouts, cauliflower and the like. As such, they share unique health benefits due to their rich concentration of glucosinolates. Regular intake of these phytochemicals is associated with a reduced risk of several cancers.

## How to buy it

The bags of shredded kale I come across in the supermarkets often taste lacklustre to me. So when it's in season, which is basically throughout the winter months, I'm always on the look out to pick up the ultra fresh leaves from the local market, farm shop or my favourite green grocers.

## How to cook it

Kale's hardy leaves take longer to cook than other greens, and unlike most other veg, it tastes better when it's well cooked. It can be steamed or simmered in some stock, whilst tougher leaves work well in soups and stews. And don't hold back on bold flavours, such as soy sauce, shallots, garlic, ginger or lemon juice.

## Pan-fried kale with garlic and anchovy butter

Whilst kale is so nutritious it is a bit like medicine, I don't think it should actually taste like medicine. Here's my attempt to change that.

Serves 4

300 g (12 oz) curly kale, shredded
20 g (¾ oz) butter
2 tbsp extra virgin olive oil
4 anchovy fillets, finely chopped
2 garlic cloves, crushed
¼ tsp dried chilli flakes
Black pepper

Steam the kale until well cooked ▇ Meanwhile, combine all the other ingredients, using a fork to mash down the butter ▇ Heat the mixture in a large pan. Add the cooked kale and sauté for 1 minute, just enough time for the kale to absorb the flavours ▇ Serve immediately.

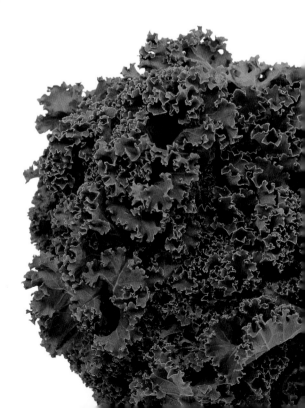

# Courgettes (Zucchini)

Courgettes are a no-frills, low-maintenance kind of vegetable, and that's what I like about them. I'd rather we ate more of these and other common-or-garden vegetables than fuss about the latest insanely expensive superfood craze.

## Why you should be eating it

Courgettes offer up a smattering of vitamins and minerals including a decent bit of vitamin C. And tucking in to a generous serving would make a worthy contribution toward the daily recommended intake for this particular vitamin. It's a pretty useful nutrient to be getting enough of, too, acting as an important antioxidant that helps protect the body against the damaging effects of free radicals. But there's more to vitamin C than just that, amongst other things playing a role in the production of collagen, which keeps connective tissue healthy in skin, cartilage and bone.

One of the unsung benefits of eating more veggies is the role they can play in maintaining a healthy weight. Courgettes are a perfect example of a low energy density food. The very type of foods we should favour to help fend off excess weight gain. With a high fibre and water content, courgettes are extremely low in fat and contain no hidden sugars. That means they'll fill us up yet only provide a small amount of calories. And in complete contrast to some faddy diets that scrimp on essential nutrients such as vitamins and minerals as much as they do calories, eating more fruits and veggies ensures an optimal intake of the vast array of beneficial plant compounds that help reduce the risk of a plethora of health problems.

## How to buy it

Aim to source your courgettes as fresh as possible. Small, firm courgettes are likely to pack the most flavour.

## How to cook it

Courgettes can be simply steamed, roasted, stir-fried, used in casseroles and stews, or they make for more unusual crudités. But in my opinion they're never better than cooked Mediterranean-style, with tomatoes, onions, garlic and fresh basil.

## Baked courgettes with mint, garlic and lemon

This veg side dish offers a welcome break from the customary steamed carrots and broccoli.

### Serves 4

4 medium courgettes (zucchini)
2 tbsp extra virgin olive oil
2 garlic cloves, crushed
Finely grated zest and juice of 1 unwaxed lemon
1 handful of mint leaves, finely chopped
Sea salt

Slice the courgettes lengthways as thinly as you can. Gently toss with the olive oil and garlic ▨ Arrange the courgettes on a baking tray and bake in a preheated oven at 200°C/400°F/gas mark 6 for about 15 minutes, until tender ▨ Remove from the oven and scatter with the lemon juice and zest, mint and a pinch of sea salt ▨ Can be served hot or left to marinate and eaten cold.

# Puy lentils

Listen up. Lentils are not just food for vegetarians. Meat-eaters would do well to get in on the act, too.

## Why you should be eating it

No prizes for knowing that lentils are full of fibre. And fibre's not just there to keep things regular, with the high level of soluble fibre in lentils assisting in lowering cholesterol levels. That, paired with a favourable effect on blood sugar control, suggests regular inclusion in the diet of lentils and pulses generally, might help reduce the risk of developing chronic health problems such as heart disease and diabetes, especially in the context of a good all-round healthy diet, a bit of exercise and maintaining a healthy body weight.

Think protein. Think iron. Chances are it conjures up images of a nice juicy steak. But lentils fit the bill, too, providing good levels of both nutrients, minus the saturated fat, of course.

As for the iron, that comes in the form of 'non-haem' iron and consequently is not absorbed as efficiently as the 'haem' iron found in meat. But, accompanying a lentil dish with vitamin C-rich foods, such as tomatoes, peppers or green leafy veg, will help the body absorb the iron more efficiently.

## How to buy it

Aside from their health benefits, lentils are cheap as chips, especially when compared with the high cost of decent quality meat.

You can either buy them in their dried form or for pure quickness and simplicity you can get them pre-cooked in a tin, but opt for the ones without added salt or sugar.

## How to cook it

Lentils are generally easier and quicker to prepare than other dried beans as they don't need lengthy pre-soaking. They make a great accompaniment to meat or fish dishes, and can work really well in salads.

# Puy lentil, red wine and mushroom casserole

I reckon this is as heart-warming as just about any meat-based dish you care to mention. And goes great with the Leek and Mustard Mash (see page 42) for bonus comfort food points.

Serves 4

250 g (9 oz) puy lentils
3 garlic cloves, crushed
300 ml (½ pt) red wine
50 ml (2 fl oz) low salt soy sauce
1 tsp dried thyme
500 g (1 lb) carrots, scrubbed (peel them if using non-organic) and thickly sliced
2 tbsp extra virgin olive oil
500 g (1 lb) open capped mushrooms, thickly sliced
1 medium onion, thinly sliced
1 bay leaf
100 g (4 oz) cashew nuts, ground to a fine powder
Black pepper

Bring the lentils to the boil along with the crushed garlic, wine, soy sauce, thyme, carrots and 300 ml (½ pint) of water. Cover and simmer until the lentils and carrots are tender, 30-40 minutes ■ Heat the oil in a large heavy-based pan and add the mushrooms, onion and bay leaf and gently cook until soft. Pour in the cooked lentils, carrots and all the cooking liquor and stir until thoroughly mixed ■ Meanwhile add a couple of tablespoons of water to the cashew nut powder and stir to ensure there are no lumps. Add this to the lentil and mushroom casserole, stir and bring to a gentle simmer. Check the seasoning and serve.

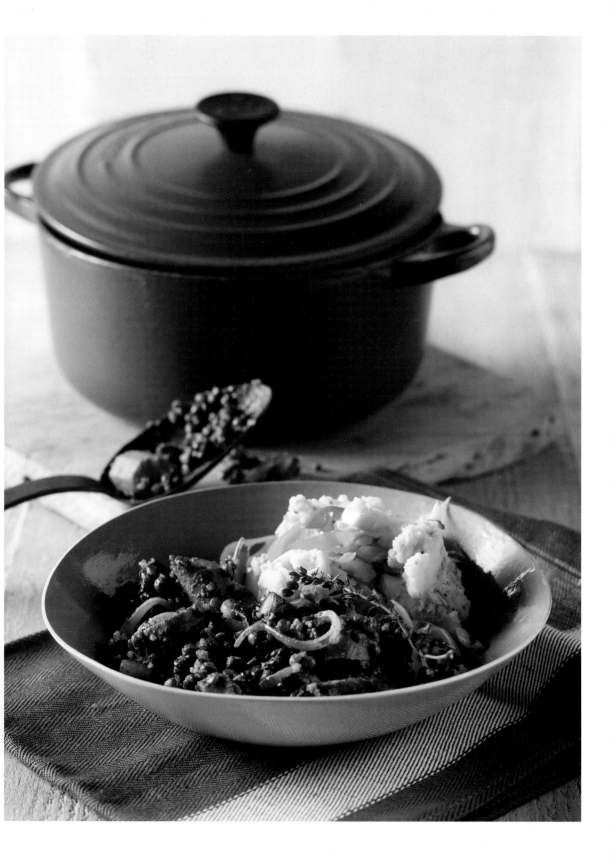

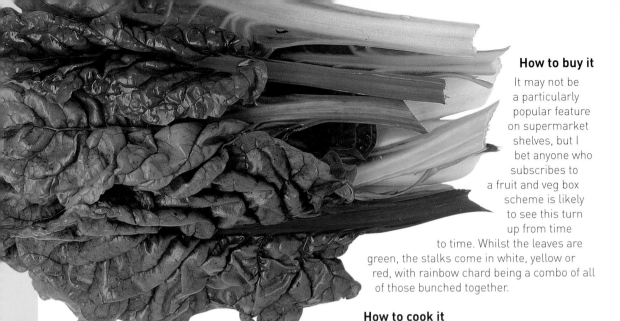

## How to buy it

It may not be a particularly popular feature on supermarket shelves, but I bet anyone who subscribes to a fruit and veg box scheme is likely to see this turn up from time to time. Whilst the leaves are green, the stalks come in white, yellow or red, with rainbow chard being a combo of all of those bunched together.

## How to cook it

Chard is good steamed or sautéed, as well as added to soups and stews. Chard leaves can happily be used in place of spinach in cooked dishes, taking just a bit longer to cook. Don't throw the stalks away, they're proper tasty, too, but do need a longer cooking time. If the stalks are really chunky I cook them separately from the leaves.

# Swiss chard

In case you hadn't guessed already, I'm on a bit of a mission to get people eating more of the green leafy stuff.

### Why you should be eating it

Chard contains bountiful amounts of carotenoids. These are the yellow, orange and red pigments found in plants and diets containing lots of carotenoid-rich fruit and veggies are associated with a reduced risk of heart disease and cancer. Chard is especially rich in two particular carotenoids called lutein and zeaxanthin, which it turns out are also present in the retina and lenses of the eyes. And it looks likely that diets rich in these two beneficial plant compounds may protect eye health by helping to reduce the risk of age-related macular degeneration and cataracts.

With chard, you also get a whole lot more thrown into the bargain. This includes a combo of the under-rated bone friendly nutrients vitamin K and magnesium. And there's plenty more to be said for getting enough magnesium, too. Whilst deficiency is rare, lowish intakes are not all that uncommon. Bad news bearing in mind it's needed for loads of different reactions to take place in the body, including helping make energy from our food.

Did I mention vitamin C? It's got a good bit of that in it, too.

## Toasted sesame Swiss chard

Proof that there's more to greens than soggy cabbage!

### Serves 4

900 g (2 lb) Swiss chard
2 tbsp groundnut oil
2 garlic cloves, finely chopped
Black pepper
2 tsp low salt soy sauce
1 tsp sesame oil
1 tbsp sesame seeds, toasted

Take the chard leaves off the stalks, finely shred the leaves and stalks – keep them separate ▧ Get a wok hot and pour in the groundnut oil. Add the stalks and stir-fry for 3-4 minutes until they begin to soften. Add the garlic and leaves and mix. Season with black pepper and stir-fry until the leaves have wilted and the stalks are soft ▧ Toss in the soy sauce, sesame oil and sesame seeds and serve.

# Onions

It's not just brightly coloured fruits and veg that do you good. Some of their pasty-looking counterparts do a pretty good job of keeping us in top-notch health, too.

## Why you should be eating it

Onions are a rich source of flavonoids, a diverse range of compounds ubiquitous in plant foods. And there's a burgeoning interest amongst researchers into the potential health benefits of these plant substances, notably in relation to protection against heart disease. Of the flavonoids, onion is particularly plentiful in quercetin, which appears to have antioxidant and anti-inflammatory activity in experimental studies, although quite how this translates from the lab to real life humans is up for debate. Foods containing quercetin may even possess cancer-protective properties notably against lung cancer risk, although the evidence for this is pretty sketchy and limited at present.

Amongst onions' fine array of phytochemicals are organosulphur compounds, similar to those found in garlic. Indeed, consumption of allium vegetables, of which onion is one, are a likely protective component of the diet against the risk of stomach cancer.

Onions are also a plentiful source of prebiotics. This is a type of fibre that resists digestion but provides a bountiful food source for our beneficial gut bacteria, stimulating their growth. Not only does that spell good news for intestinal health, but other suggested benefits of prebiotics include increased absorption of minerals such as calcium from the diet and enhanced immune system function.

## How to buy it

Onions are cheap, plentiful and store well. And with such abundant home-grown produce, I see no good reason not to buy local.

## How to cook it

If you're into cooking fresh food from scratch, onions have to be about one of the most basic staple ingredients I can think of and form the basis of many a heart-warming soup, casserole, curry or tomato sauce to name but a few. Raw spring onions and red onions are especially good for pepping up salads, sandwiches and fillings for pitta bread.

## Onion gravy

I don't care what anyone says, gravy out of a packet isn't a patch on the stuff you make from scratch. Just don't rush the onions...

Serves 4

50 g (2 oz) unsalted butter
2-3 medium onions, thinly sliced
25 g (1 oz) plain (all-purpose) flour
500 ml (1 pt) hot vegetable stock (use 3 tsp of powder)
150 ml (¼ pt) red wine
1 tbsp tomato purée (tomato paste)
2 tsp Worcestershire sauce
1 tsp dried thyme or 1 tbsp of fresh
Black pepper

Melt the butter and gently soften the sliced onions until they're practically melting. Allow a good amount of time for this, 20 minutes or so ▦ Once they're soft and a little brown at the edges (where the natural sugars have caramelized), add the plain flour, stir through and cook for a few moments. Pour in the hot stock and wine, stirring continuously until the sauce thickens ▦ Once the gravy has thickened, add the tomato purée, Worcestershire sauce, dried or fresh thyme and freshly ground black pepper. Simmer with the odd bubble breaking on the surface for 30 minutes, giving it the occasional stir to stop it sticking ▦ Pour into a warmed gravy jug and serve.

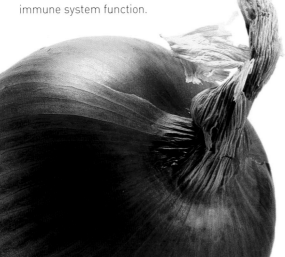

# Fast food

If there's one thing food has to be nowadays, it's fast. Convenience rules and I can fully understand why. When we're out and about fast food is available at every turn. We're surrounded by the stuff and it starts to look pretty attractive if you don't have time to prepare intricate meals from scratch (especially after a long day at work). Like it or not, this isn't likely to change anytime soon. You only need look at the sprawl of fast food outlets or the supermarket floorspace given over to ready-meals to see that we've fallen for convenience food hook, line and sinker. I can't see much point in getting too moralistic about it all – after all, convenience is really important to most people. So I reckon it's a whole lot better to embrace the fast food idea, but with a twist. In short, fast food that's good for you.

Here's the drill. I worked out it takes about 30 minutes for me to phone up the local takeaway, place the order, go collect it, drive home, serve up and get comfy to eat. So that's the criteria I'm using for fast food here – the 30 minute rule. And the recipes in this chapter should be achievable in less than that. Of course, the real deal breaker is the fact that the grub served up here is actually doing you some good.

At the end of the day, it's all about priorities. If you're just looking to fill a hole as quickly as possible, with no regard to whether it's doing you any good or not, then the recipes in this chapter probably aren't for you. Stick to your take-outs. But if you do care about what you're putting inside you, this is all achievable if you can find a few extra minutes each day. And if you're prepared to do that, read on!

# Mushrooms

It's the brightly coloured fruits and veggies that steal the health plaudits and hog the limelight, leaving their more washed-out looking counterparts in the dark. But I reckon one of the pasty brigade, the mushroom, is a bit of a hidden gem.

## Why you should be eating it

Of the more conventional nutrients, mushrooms provide a fine selection of B-vitamins, which amongst other things, are important for helping release energy from food and the trace mineral selenium, which folk in some countries generally aren't getting enough of, despite growing awareness of its potentially important role in helping protect against cancer.

There have been lots of bold claims made about the medicinal properties of mushrooms, notably for their immune enhancing and anti-cancer properties, likely to be due to their polysaccharide compounds. And in recent years, researchers have begun to accumulate some evidence in support of this.

Whilst a lot of this has focussed on the higher profile 'exotic' mushrooms like shiitake and maitake, common-or-garden mushrooms may be in with a shout, too, with some emerging research suggesting possible protective effects of regular mushroom consumption against the development of breast cancer. Interesting stuff, but it's very early days and nowhere near enough research has been carried out to more fully understand how mushrooms might be used to improve our health.

## How to buy it

Fresh mushrooms abound and are widely available. The more exotic mushrooms, such as shiitake, are increasingly available both in fresh and dried forms.

## How to cook it

Mushrooms are really versatile and work well in just about anything from salads, to stir-fries, to soups and casseroles.

# Mushroom and water chestnut stir-fry

This has got to be loads better than what the local take-away is dishing up. If you like your sauces a tad sweeter, by all means add some honey to taste.

### Serves 4

3 tbsp groundnut oil
3 garlic cloves, finely chopped
2 red chillies, deseeded and finely chopped
2 lemon grass sticks, outer leaves discarded
    and finely shredded
2½ cm (1 in) long piece of ginger, peeled and grated
500 g (1 lb) chestnut mushrooms, thickly sliced
1 x 225 g (8 oz) tin of water chestnuts, sliced
150 g (5 oz) spinach, coarsely shredded
3–4 tbsp low salt soy sauce
3–4 tsp dry sherry or rice wine vinegar

Heat a wok until smoking. Pour in the oil, garlic, chilli, lemon grass and ginger and stir-fry for 15 seconds or so but not so long that everything goes crisp ■ Add the mushrooms and water chestnuts and fry until they start to become golden and soft ■ Throw in the spinach leaves and the dish should be ready once the leaves have wilted and are still vivid green ■ Add the soy sauce and dry sherry or rice wine vinegar according to your taste and serve on warmed plates with noodles.

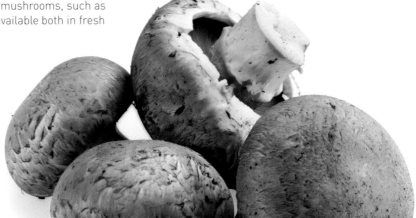

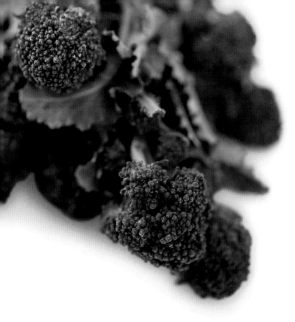

# Purple sprouting broccoli

To me, purple sprouting broccoli represents everything that's exciting about seasonal food. As it's only around for a relatively short chunk of time, I look forward to getting my hands on the stuff.

### Why you should be eating it

Broccoli is a member of the cruciferous family of vegetables, along with such notable others as cabbage, Brussels sprouts and cauliflower. There's a flurry of interest amongst researchers looking at how regular consumption of these veggies might help protect against the development of various common cancers and possibly even heart disease, too.

What marks them out for special attention is their uniquely high levels of glucosinolates. Okay, here come all the big fancy words. Hang in there. These clever plant chemicals get broken down into active compounds called isothiocyanates. Broccoli is especially rich in a particular type called sulforaphane, which appears to discourage the development of cancer in a number of different ways, although more research in humans still needs to be done to better understand this.

Of course, being all dark, green and with a bit of leafiness going on, you'd expect there to be a lot of other good stuff in there, too. So there is, with broccoli containing a good hit of bone-building vitamin K along with a smidgen of calcium and magnesium for good measure. And that's before we even mention a bunch of antioxidants, such as vitamin C and carotenoids.

### How to buy it

Seize the seasonal stuff from late winter through to late spring, trying to bag ultra-fresh and locally grown where you can find it.

### How to cook it

If you've landed some really fresh broccoli, then keep it simple. Steam until just tender and drizzle with extra virgin olive oil. Alternatively, it makes for a great addition to a pasta dish or stir-fried with garlic, chilli and a splash of soy sauce.

## Purple sprouting broccoli and tuna pasta

When time is tight, out comes the pasta and tuna. That's life. But here we've ramped up the health credentials a notch or two.

### Serves 4

500 g (1 lb) wholewheat Penne or Fusilli pasta
1 kg (2 lb) purple sprouting broccoli, cut into bite sized pieces
2 large garlic cloves, finely chopped
2 x 200 g (7 oz) tin (150 g/5 oz drained weight) of tuna in spring water, drained and flaked
2 x 50 g (2 oz) tin (30 g/1 oz) drained weight) anchovy fillets in extra virgin olive oil (reserve the oil), chopped
Handful of toasted pumpkin and sunflower seeds
Black pepper
Small pinch of chilli flakes

Bring a large pan of water to the boil and cook the pasta according to instructions ▪ Place a steamer above the pasta and steam the broccoli for 5 minutes until tender ▪ Meanwhile fry the garlic in 1 tablespoon of the reserved anchovy oil until lightly golden. Add the flaked tuna and chopped anchovies and mix well, fry until heated through ▪ Once cooked, drain the pasta and stir through the tuna mix, broccoli and toasted seeds. Season with plenty of black pepper, a pinch of chilli flakes and serve.

# Mussels

One of the things I like about shellfish is that it provides abundant amounts of some of the nutrients that tend to be low in typical modern diets. Sort of like the missing piece of a jigsaw puzzle.

## Why you should be eating it

Mussels offer a top-notch protein source, whilst being low in saturated fat. But they're not an entirely low fat food, containing appreciable amounts of omega-3 fatty acids, just like the kinds found in oily fish, but at relatively lower levels. And on the whole our intake of these 'good' fats has declined. This is a pity bearing in mind the myriad of health benefits they offer for cardiovascular health, for the structure and function of the brain, not to mention their anti-inflammatory properties.

The same is true of selenium, which mussels provide in plentiful amounts. Particularly relevant in the context of concerns is that intake of this trace mineral has declined in the typical diet of some nations in recent decades. And it's a big-time player, involved in our antioxidant defences, thyroid function, immunity and reproductive health. There's also a big debate as to whether our low intakes may be increasing the risk of cancer.

And they're not short of another mineral or two either, containing substantial amounts of zinc, iron and iodine. Nor vitamins for that matter, providing good levels of folate, along with exceptional amounts of vitamin B12, partners in crime when it comes to lowering levels of homocysteine in the blood, high levels of which are implicated in heart disease.

## How to buy it

Rope-grown or hand-gathered represent the more environmentally sustainable options.

And when it comes to shellfish, I'm much happier buying them from a reputable source when they're really fresh, and cooking them as quickly as possible.

## How to cook it

It goes without saying that it's important to take care with storing, preparing and cooking mussels to avoid an unwelcome bout of food poisoning. No one needs that.

# Thai style mussels

A real meal in minutes.

### Serves 2 (or 4 as a starter)

1 kg (2 lb) live mussels
6 spring onions (scallions), roughly chopped
1 lemon grass, outer leaves removed and roughly chopped
5 cm (2 in) piece of ginger, peeled and roughly chopped
2 garlic cloves, roughly chopped
2 red chillies, deseeded and finely chopped
Large bunch of fresh coriander (cilantro), roughly chopped
1 tbsp extra virgin olive oil
1 x 400 ml (14 fl oz) tin of coconut milk
1 tbsp fish sauce
Juice of 1 lime

Put the mussels into a bowl of cold, clean water and spend a little time going through them, one by one, making sure you discard the ones that refuse to close the instant you give them a tap or those with cracked shells. Give them a good scrub, cleaning off any barnacles, mud and removing their beards (the long straggly hairs) ▦ Place the roughly chopped spring onions, lemon grass, ginger, garlic, red chillies and most of the coriander into a blender and whizz to a coarse paste ▦ Heat the oil in a large pan. Fry the paste for 3 minutes over a moderate heat. Add the coconut milk, fish sauce and lime juice and bring to a simmer. Add the mussels, cover with a tight fitting lid, and cook over a high heat for 3-4 minutes until all the mussels are open – discard any that aren't ▦ Serve immediately in a bowl with the mussels covered in the coconut liquor, topped with some chopped coriander, and have plenty of crusty wholemeal bread at the ready to mop up all those lovely juices.

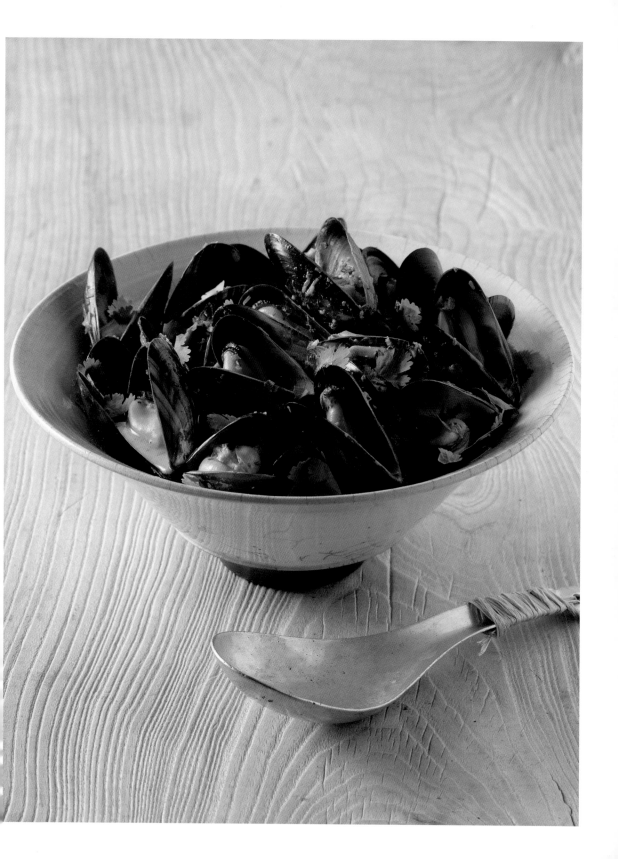

# White fish

With all the huff and puff about oily fish, white fish has taken a bit of a back seat. But there is a whole lot more to fish than just omega-3's, making white fish quite the catch.

## Why you should be eating it

White fish provides an exceptional source of protein, comparable with meat, but with the added bonus of very low levels of saturated fat.

It also provides really useful amounts of nutrients that are not always easily or reliably available from other foods. Top of the list is selenium. There are concerns that people in some countries just aren't getting ideal amounts of selenium needed for optimal health, which may be leaving us vulnerable to various health problems, notably an increased risk of cancer.

Although the evidence is inconsistent, fish consumption has been related to a lower incidence of colorectal cancer. Whilst this may be down to the beneficial omega-3 fats found in oily fish, or the fact that people who eat a lot of fish might eat less meat, it could also be partly due to factors such as its selenium content.

White fish also comes up trumps with good levels of iodine, important for thyroid function, and B-vitamins, notably B12.

## How to buy it

Think sustainability. Fish stocks are rapidly dwindling. Whilst it's a complicated business, one of the simplest things you can do is keep your eyes peeled for the Marine Stewardship Council logo or choose less exploited fish, such as pollack or gurnard.

## How to cook it

Bake it, grill it, pan-fry or poach it. As much as I hate to say it, if it comes deep-fried in batter, you'll be undoing its health benefits quicker than you can say mushy peas. And remember that the secret to cooking white fish is not to completely overcook it.

## Grilled white fish with coriander pesto

This is fast food at its healthiest and perfect if you've endured a late one at the office and are in need of a quick fix. The time it takes to grill the fish gives you just enough time to rustle up the coriander pesto and a quick green salad.

### Serves 2

2 x 150 g (5 oz) white fish (such as pollack) fillets
1 tbsp extra virgin olive oil
Sea salt and black pepper

FOR THE CORIANDER PESTO
50 g (2 oz) fresh coriander (cilantro), roughly chopped and tough stalks removed
2 garlic cloves, crushed
4 tbsp pine nuts
A pinch of dried chilli flakes
2 tbsp extra virgin olive oil

Kick things off by brushing the fish with olive oil and season. Cook under a hot grill for 10-12 minutes or until cooked through ▪ For the pesto, place all the ingredients except the oil into a food processor. Blend, adding the oil bit by bit, until you reach the desired paste-like consistency ▪ When the fish is cooked, serve immediately with a lovely big dollop of the coriander pesto and a fresh green salad.

# Asparagus

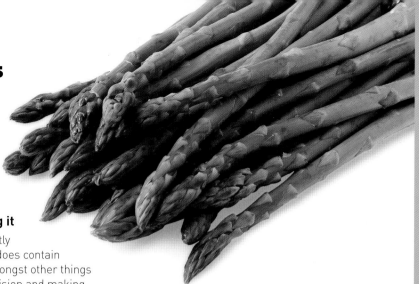

I only eat asparagus in spring when it's bang in season. And I definitely make the most of it during those couple of months.

### Why you should be eating it

Whilst asparagus is not exactly a nutritional heavyweight, it does contain useful amounts of folate, amongst other things important for normal cell division and making healthy red blood cells, also for helping to keep levels of homocysteine in check, raised levels of which appear to be an independent risk factor for heart disease.

But as ever with fruits and veggies, we can't explain away all the health benefits from looking just at the conventional vitamins and minerals. Asparagus is one of a number of foods that contains appreciable amounts of prebiotics. You've probably already heard of probiotics, the 'good' bacteria that you find in 'live' yoghurts or yoghurt drinks. Well, prebiotics are different in as much as they're a type of fibre that selectively encourages the growth of the beneficial bacteria that are already in the digestive tract.

As well as promoting a healthy digestive system, other potential benefits or prebiotics include improving the absorption of minerals such as calcium, enhancing immunity, possibly even cancer-protective properties and cholesterol lowering effects.

### How to buy it

Asparagus at its best will be firm, have lovely green spears and tight tips. Go for the younger, thinner spears when you can.

### How to cook it

Asparagus is grown in sandy soil and there's nothing worse than crunching on the gritty bits that can get caught in the tips, so be sure to give it a really good wash under cold water. Steam, boil or grill it.

## Asparagus simply

When you've got some top-notch quality ingredients, sometimes the best thing you can do is not mess about with them too much. Less is more and all that.

### Per person

8 asparagus spears
25 g (1 oz) unsalted butter
A few chives, finely chopped
Freshly ground black pepper

Wash the asparagus gently. Take each spear at the base and gently bend it so that it snaps, which gets rid of the woody bit 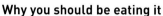 Bring a large frying pan or sauté pan, with just enough water to cover the spears, to the boil. Place the spears in and simmer them until tender when pierced with the point of a knife. This should take about 3-5 minutes (depending on thickness and age) ▧ As the spears are simmering, gently melt the butter in a small pan ▧ To serve, drain the asparagus and arrange in a criss-cross pattern on some warmed plates. Pour over the melted butter. Sprinkle over the chives and black pepper.

Asparagus is also delicious served with a poached egg – the yolk makes a fantastically simple sauce for the spears – and also works well with scrambled eggs and wholemeal toast for a posh take on a fast food favourite.

# Avocado

Avocados, with their high fat content, are eyed with suspicion by many people who've adopted the ultra low fat mindset. Give me 5 minutes and I'll see if I can persuade you otherwise.

## Why you should be eating it

Undoubtedly avocados are a proper fatty of a food and inevitably that means they comes with more than their fair share of calories, too. Not the sort of food that you'd want to be eating by the bucket load. But I reckon it's time we started thinking a bit differently about fat and focus on the quality of fat in the diet, not just the quantity. The predominant fat in avocados is of the monounsaturated type, a healthy fat that can assist in lowering 'bad' LDL cholesterol levels, especially if it replaces the more cholesterol-raising saturated fats.

And with that thought in mind, we might even begin to view avocados as a heart-friendly food. As well as providing a good dose of healthful oils, they're awash with other cardio-protective nutrients, such as the antioxidants vitamin C and E and blood pressure regulating potassium. So as unfeasible as it sounds for a high fat food, avocados fit the bill quite nicely when it comes to cardio-protection.

Just like other fruits and veggies, avocados contain a plentiful array of other nutrients and bioactive compounds including the carotenoid lutein that may play a role in maintaining eye health as we age. And adding some avocado to your salad should help to increase the absorption of healthful carotenoids (the likes of beta carotene, lutein and lycopene) from the other salad veggies. Carotenoids are fat soluble and the presence of fats in avocado gives a helping hand in promoting their uptake into the body (although a splash of olive oil in a dressing would likely do the job just fine, too).

## How to buy it

Bullet-hard, under-ripe avocados always disappoint, so be on the look-out for properly ripe avocados, which will be slightly soft when given a squeeze.

## How to cook it

This is a food that you don't need to cook, making it an ultimate convenience food. Guacamole is the obvious choice. But avocado is never better than when added to salads and also works a treat in sandwiches, pitta bread or mashed up and spread on toast.

## Guacamole

I'm never sure about that strange mass produced homogenous stuff you can buy pre-made in plastic tubs. It's not guacamole as I know it. The key to this recipe are properly soft, ripe avocados.

### Serves 4

3 ripe avocados
Juice of ½ a lime
6 spring onions (scallions), finely chopped
8 cherry tomatoes, finely chopped
2 mild fresh chillies, deseeded and finely chopped
2 tbsp fresh coriander (cilantro), finely chopped
Sea salt and black pepper

Scoop the flesh from the avocado and add it to a bowl with the lime juice, spring onions, cherry tomatoes, chilli and coriander ■ Roughly mash (a fork works fine). Season with a pinch of sea salt and black pepper.

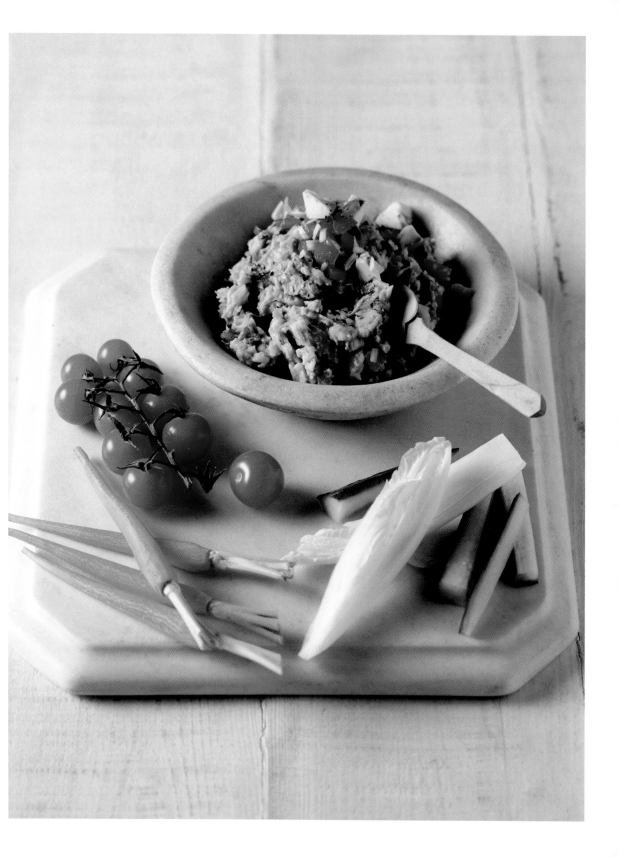

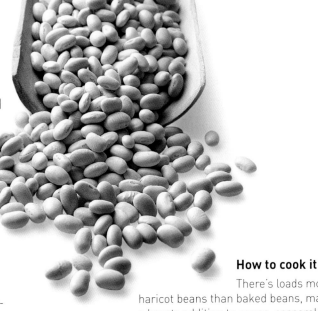

# Haricot (Navy) beans

We're talking the stuff of baked beans fame here. That I, and just about every other kid I ever knew, grew up feasting on these is testament to the fact that beans can be a palatable food and not just the stuff healthfood cranks eat.

## Why you should be eating it

Brimming with protein, fibre and slow-release carbohydrates, haricot beans offer a prescription for good health. No surprises then to uncover that pulses are an archetypal heart-friendly food, with the ability to help reduce levels of cholesterol in the blood, and consequently the risk of heart disease.

Baked beans are famed for their, what shall we say, wind-inducing nature. And that's likely to be to do with their high level of fibre, including a type of indigestible starch called resistant starch, which the bacteria in our large intestine have a whale of a time fermenting. But in so doing, a lot of good substances are produced, notably short-chain fatty acids that have a positive effect on the health of the colon.

And whilst dietary fibre doesn't possess the glitz and glamour of the more heavily marketed 'superfoods', let's not forget that it does some important stuff, such as helping to prevent constipation and lends a hand in warding off more serious conditions affecting the digestive tract like diverticulitis and bowel cancer.

## How to buy it

Baked beans are a great food, just watch out for undesirable levels of added sugar and salt. Alternatively, you can buy tinned haricot beans just as they are, again opting for ones without the unnecessary addition of sugar or salt. And of course, having them out of a tin isn't compulsory, in which case buy them dried and pre-soak and cook accordingly.

## How to cook it

There's loads more to haricot beans than baked beans, making a hearty addition to soups, casseroles, salads or homemade chilli.

## Homemade baked beans

It's not as convenient as cracking open a tin, but if you're a fan of baked beans, I reckon this is worth the extra effort.

### Serves 4

1 tbsp of olive oil
1 medium red onion, finely chopped
1 garlic clove, crushed
½ tsp ground cumin
½ tsp ground coriander
½ tsp paprika
¼ tsp cayenne pepper
½ tsp dried oregano
1 x 410 g (14 oz) tin of haricot (navy) beans
1 x 400 g (14 oz) tin of chopped tomatoes
1 tbsp tomato purée (tomato paste)
1 tbsp tamari soy sauce
1 tsp blackstrap molasses

Heat the oil in a saucepan and gently sauté the onions and garlic for 5 minutes until the onions are translucent ■ Add the cumin, coriander, paprika, cayenne pepper and oregano and stir well ■ Add the beans, tomatoes, tomato purée, soy sauce and molasses and gently simmer for 10 minutes.

# Sesame seeds

Not the most thrilling of foods, granted, but just like a caterpillar, sesame seeds can transform into something special (that's actually tahini, not a butterfly). It involves blitzing them into a paste, a bit like peanut butter (please never attempt this with a caterpillar).

## Why you should be eating it

Sesame seed's number one claim to fame is their very respectable calcium content. And no prizes for knowing that calcium is needed for strong bones. But calcium is good for health in other ways, too, possibly helping to lower elevated blood pressure, along with a bit of evidence to suggest it may help to protect against certain types of cancer such as colon and breast cancer, although more research is needed on this to be sure.

Despite their diminutive size, sesame seeds have some big heart-health credentials. First up, they contain high levels of cardio-protective healthy fats of the monounsaturated and polyunsaturated kind. And like nuts and seeds generally, they're also packed with cholesterol-lowering phytosterols, just like the active ingredient added to cholesterol-lowering margarines, albeit in smaller amounts.

Whilst flaxseeds are generally acknowledged to be the richest dietary source of plant compounds called lignans, sesame seeds appear to be a pretty decent source, too. This is of interest insofar as researchers are looking in to whether lignans may help to protect against hormone-related diseases like breast cancer.

## How to buy it

No insider knowledge needed here. You can pick sesame seeds up in just about any health food shop or supermarket. And there's also tahini, which for the uninitiated is a bit like peanut butter, but made from roasted sesame seeds instead.

## How to cook it

To add a nutty vibe, toasted sesame seeds are good tossed on savoury dishes such as stir-fries or salads. As for tahini, it's most definitely not just the preserve of health food cranks, but an integral aspect of Middle Eastern cuisine, featuring in classic dishes such as hummus and halva, both of which are pretty easy to knock up from scratch at home.

# Spice-topped hummus

With the welcome addition of this spice-laden topping, my bet is that once you've sampled this little number, you'll find it hard to go back to the mass produced stuff.

Serves 4

FOR THE SPICY TOPPING
1 tbsp extra virgin olive oil
1 large red onion, halved and finely sliced
1 tsp ground cumin
1 tsp ground coriander
1 tsp paprika
½ tsp black onion seeds
½ tsp turmeric
½ tsp ground ginger
½ tsp ground cinnamon
¼ tsp ground nutmeg
Black pepper
A pinch of ground cloves
A pinch of ground cardamom
1 tbsp tamari soy sauce
1 tsp clear honey

FOR THE HUMMUS
500 g (1½ lb) cooked chickpeas (approximately 2 cans)
2 tbsp tahini
2 tbsp clear honey
6 tbsp extra virgin olive oil
Juice of 1 lemon
Zest of ½ unwaxed lemon
2 garlic cloves, crushed
2 fresh red chilli peppers, deseeded and roughly chopped
200 ml (7 fl oz) water
Sea salt and black pepper

First make the spicy topping. Heat the olive oil in a shallow frying pan. Add the red onion and gently fry for approximately 10 minutes until the onions are soft and translucent ■ Add all of the spices to the frying pan along with the tamari and the honey. Add a splash of water to prevent the spices from sticking to the pan. Continue to cook for 5 minutes ■ Remove from the heat and allow to cool ■ Put all of the ingredients for the hummus into a blender and blend until smooth. Add more water if necessary ■ Put the hummus into a large bowl and top with the spice mixture.

# Lazy Sundays

For some reason, the food I eat on Sundays is totally different from the rest of the week. It's got to be something to do with the slower pace of the day. It's more chilled-out and so is the way I prepare and eat food. I love that feeling of having quality time to cook, and when I get a Sunday like that, I make the most of it.

Breakfast never happens early and for that very reason, I'll nearly always have something more extravagant to eat than on a weekday. Armed with the Sunday paper, it's the perfect way to start the day. And no Sunday is quite complete without a proper Sunday dinner. Personally, I'm not hung up on it being an overly traditional affair. I'm quite happy to play around with it, maybe cooking a whole chicken with curry spices or roasting a tray of more unusual veggies. With some good-quality, properly reared meat and a big emphasis on the veg, this can be as healthy as it is hearty.

But Sundays aren't all about cooked breakfasts and full-on roast dinners. After all that indulgence, come Sunday evening, I'm mostly happy to prepare some tasty home-made snack food or a hearty soup and kick back and watch a film. And, all in all, that's probably the meal I enjoy the most. So, here are the recipes. Book Sunday off now and enjoy it!

# Beef

Roast beef. Mmmm. When it comes to health, red meat has a tarnished reputation, but it's not all bad news and I for one won't be striking roast beef off the menu anytime soon.

## Why you should be eating it

Beef is abundant in a range of nutrients, notably protein, zinc, vitamin B12 and iron. Whilst you can happily get these nutrients from a whole range of other foods, there are few individual foods that provide all of these nutrients at quite the same levels and in quite such well absorbed forms.

Zinc is involved in all sorts of reactions in the body and plays an important role in growth, tissue repair and healing, immunity, and reproductive and skin health. And as it happens, zinc is generally better absorbed from meat than from foods such as cereals and pulses (although they can still provide a good source, too).

The same applies to iron, which in red meat comes in the form of 'haem' iron and is really well absorbed compared to iron from plant foods. And getting sufficient iron in the diet is particularly important for teenage girls and women of child-bearing age as their requirements are generally higher.

But a few words of warning. There's no doubting that red meats such as beef are high in saturated fat. And too much of that is linked to increased cholesterol levels and heart disease. So the emphasis should be on leaner cuts. The other problem we can't ignore is the link between red meat consumption and an increased risk of colon cancer. So moderation is definitely the name of the game.

## How to buy it

There's a world of difference between good-quality lean cuts of beef and cheap, fatty, heavily processed meat. It goes without saying that the former represents an altogether healthier choice.

## How to cook it

Cuts of beef come in all shapes and sizes and this will determine how you go about cooking it. But one thing worth knowing is that high temperature cooking that leads to charring or burning of the meat generates harmful chemicals linked with an increased risk of cancer. Barbecuing, grilling or frying being the worst offenders. In contrast, a longer cooking time at a lower temperature, think stews and casseroles, produces far fewer of these potentially harmful chemicals.

## Pot roast beef and ale

Stick this on to cook. Batten down the hatches. Find your favourite spot on the sofa. Get snug. Watch a film. Doze off. Wake up. Serve.

### Serves 4

25 g (1 oz) unsalted butter
1 tbsp olive oil
1 kg (2 lb) rolled brisket of beef
4 small carrots, scrubbed and cut into
    5 cm (2 in) lengths
2 large celery sticks, cut into 5 cm (2 in) lengths
1 large onion, thickly sliced
100 g (4 oz) open-capped mushrooms, thickly sliced
1 parsnip, scrubbed and cut into 5 cm (2 in) pieces
300 ml (½ pt) light or dark ale
Small handful of thyme sprigs
2 bay leaves
1 tsp Worcestershire sauce
½ tsp English mustard
Sea salt and black pepper
1 tbsp cornflour

Preheat the oven to 150°C/300°F/gas mark 2
■ Warm the butter and olive oil in a large, ovenproof casserole dish and brown the beef on all sides. Remove the beef and replace with all the vegetables and cook over a moderate heat to lightly brown ■ Add the ale, herbs, Worcestershire sauce, mustard and seasoning and bring to a gentle boil. Place the brisket of beef gently on top of the vegetables, cover with a tight fitting lid (if you don't have one cover with foil). Cook in the oven for 2½–3 hours ■ When ready, place the beef and vegetables onto a warmed serving dish and leave to rest in a warm place for 10 minutes. Bring the remaining juices up to a boil and boil fast to reduce slightly ■ Mix the cornflour with a little water to a smooth paste and stir into the gravy, stirring constantly until it thickens. Check the seasoning and pour into a gravy jug. Carve the beef and serve with a ladle of vegetables covered in gravy.

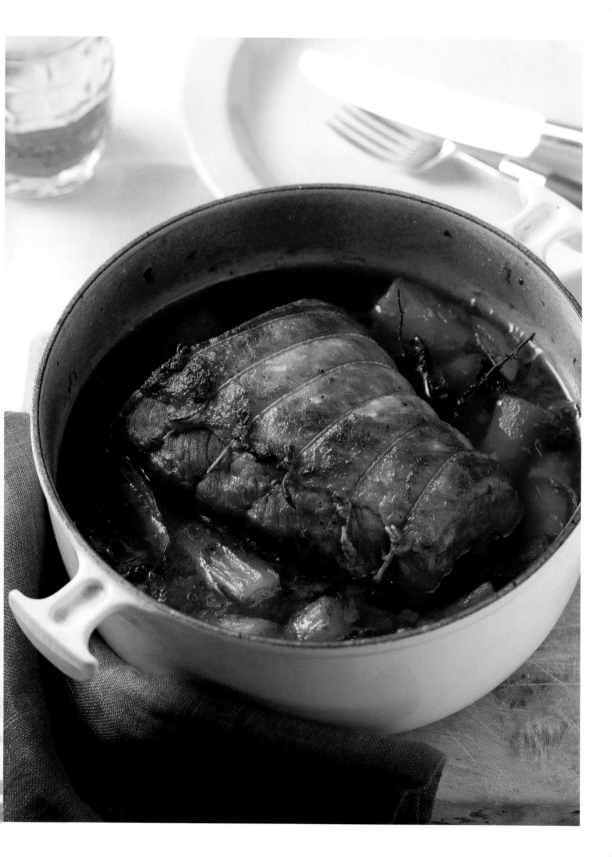

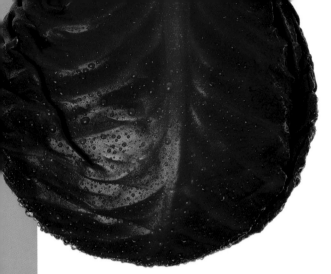

# Red cabbage

I've got two problems with cabbage, memories of bad school dinners with over-cooked, sludgy cabbage, and shredded red cabbage that comes pickled in a jar. No need. But I'm over that and reckon cabbage is deserving of a second chance.

### Why you should be eating it

We tend to think that vitamin C only comes from fruit. Stuff like oranges or kiwis. But red cabbage offers plentiful amounts of this antioxidant vitamin, along with useful amounts of fibre for digestive health.

Cabbage is also part of the wider family of cruciferous vegetables, along with other veggies such as broccoli, Brussels sprouts, cauliflower and kale. There's avid interest amongst researchers into the potential for these vegetables to reduce the risk of certain types of cancer. And that's thought to be down to their uniquely rich content of glucosinolates. But it's not the glucosinolates that do the work. Rather it's their break-down products, the bio-active isothiocyanates, that are generating big interest for their promising anti-cancer properties.

It's the brightly coloured fruits and veggies that tend to be packed full of sizeable amounts of antioxidants and phytochemicals. And this is true of red cabbage, which is loaded with beneficial plant compounds known as flavonoids, notably anthocyanins, responsible for its purple colouring. Whilst we still don't know enough about the potential health benefits of anthocyanins, they've garnered interest amongst researchers for their potential role in such diverse areas as helping to keep the aging brain functioning well, possible benefits for cardiovascular health and even cancer-preventive properties.

### How to buy it

If you can, stick with local, seasonal produce, even better if it's organic.

### How to cook it

Red cabbage is sublime when braised slowly with apples for a hearty winter vegetable dish. It's also at its rough and rugged crunchy best in home-made coleslaw or a winter salad.

## Slow-cooked red cabbage with apple

This is a great winter warmer and would be just the thing to accompany Pot Roast Beef and Ale (see page 114).

Serves 4

3 tbsp extra virgin olive oil
1 onion, finely chopped
2 garlic cloves, finely chopped
1 kg (2 lb) red cabbage, finely shredded
    (about half a large cabbage)
2 large cooking apples (such as Bramleys),
    peeled and sliced
2 tbsp maple syrup
Juice of ½ lemon
2 tbsp red wine vinegar
Black pepper
1 tbsp caraway seeds

Heat the oil in a large heavy-based pan and fry the onion and garlic gently until softened ■ Add the cabbage, apple and maple syrup and stir to bring the onions and garlic up from the bottom of the pan. Mix well. Cook gently for 10 minutes, shaking the pan occasionally to make sure nothing is sticking ■ Add the lemon juice, vinegar, pepper and caraway seeds. Cover and simmer gently for 1–1 ½ hours, shaking or stirring occasionally. Add a little water if the mixture looks a little dry. It's ready once the cabbage and apple are melt-in-the mouth soft.

# Tomato purée (Tomato paste)

It's not often that a processed version of a fresh food wins the plaudits, but tomato purée is the exception to the rule.

### Why you should be eating it

There can't be many foods that have attracted the interest of researchers as much as the tomato. And it's the stuff that gives tomatoes their red hue, lycopene, that's dominated the headlines. Whilst one or two other foods contain lycopene, tomatoes are far and away the major dietary source.

As well as acting as a powerful antioxidant, clever laboratory experiments have shown lycopene to inhibit cancer cells. Of course, just because that happens in little dishes and test tubes in a laboratory doesn't mean it will necessarily have the same effect inside us when we eat it. Whilst numerous, if not all, population-based studies have reported an association between consumption of tomatoes and a degree of protection against certain types of cancer, notably prostate cancer, the evidence is not yet conclusive.

But here's the deal-breaker. Lycopene is tightly bound up in the cellular structure of the tomato. So if you eat it raw, you don't actually absorb that much. But cooking and processing tomatoes frees-up the lycopene and makes it more 'bioavailable'. And that points to tomato purée or paste being an ideal way to bump-up lycopene intake. Even better if combined with a little bit of oil or fat at a meal, which gives a further boost to lycopene absorption.

Of course, there are loads of other beneficial nutrients and phytochemicals to be found in a tomato other than lycopene. And there's no reason to think that tomato purée won't also give you a concentrated dose of those, too.

### How to buy it

Being such a storecupboard essential, tomato purée is available far and wide and should contain nothing other than tomatoes.

### How to cook it

Tomato purée is one of those basic ingredients with all manner of culinary uses. Its full-on tomato flavour can ramp-up home-made tomato sauces and pizza toppings, casseroles, stews and soups.

## Spicy bean and tomato soup

This soup is full-on heartiness. A one-pot meal that's perfect for a Sunday evening. And if you cheat and use canned beans, it's ready in a flash, meaning you can kick back and enjoy what's left of your weekend.

### Serves 4

2 tbsp extra virgin olive oil
2 red onions, chopped
2 garlic cloves, crushed
1 celery stalk, thinly sliced
1 green (bell) pepper, chopped
1 tsp ground coriander
1 tsp ground cumin
1 tsp paprika
½ tsp dried oregano
¼ tsp dried chilli flakes (more if you like it hot)
¼ tsp cayenne pepper
1 x 410 g (14 oz) tin red kidney beans, drained
1 x 410 g (14 oz) tin black-eye beans, drained
1 x 410 g (14 oz) tin butter (lima) beans, drained
1 large jar (700 g/1½ lb) tomato passata (tomato sauce)
3 tbsp tomato purée (tomato paste)
2 tbsp tamari soy sauce
200 ml (7 fl oz) water
Black pepper to taste
Grated Cheddar cheese, to serve

Heat the olive oil in a large pan and gently fry the onions until soft ■ Add the garlic, celery and green pepper and continue to cook for a further 5 minutes, until the vegetables begin to soften ■ Add the coriander, cumin, paprika, oregano, chilli flakes and cayenne pepper and continue to cook for 2 minutes. Stir in the beans ■ Stir in the tomato passata, tomato purée, tamari and water and combine well ■ Season and simmer uncovered for 20 minutes, stirring occasionally ■ Serve just as it is, or top with some grated cheese.

# Chestnuts

When I roast chestnuts they never seem to taste as good as the ones sold by street vendors at Christmas, but this recipe is top-notch and can be cooked all year.

### Why you should be eating it

At complete odds to other nuts, chestnuts contain very little fat. Instead, they contain much higher levels of carbohydrates, and overall, have quite a different nutritional make-up. For example, they're a rich source of vitamin C. Amongst its numerous functions this vitamin acts as an important antioxidant and is involved in collagen formation making it important for healthy skin, cartilage and bone. Chestnuts also happen to be a decent source of B-vitamins, notably vitamins B6 and folate, which work together to keep blood levels of homocysteine under control, a good thing as high levels are associated with heart disease risk.

But chestnuts do have something in common with other nuts, notably the fact that they're brimming with antioxidants. In fact, they're not far off the pace of walnuts and pecans, the antioxidant heavyweights of the nut world. And for the uninitiated, antioxidants help to protect the body from the damage caused by free radicals, excessive levels of which are implicated in the development of numerous chronic diseases, not to mention the ageing process itself.

### How to buy it

When they're in season, you can buy them fresh in their shells, ideal for roasting. But if I'm using chestnuts for recipes, then I'll just cheat and go for the convenience of buying them in a jar, cooked, peeled and ready to roll.

### How to cook it

In addition to Christmassy roasted chestnuts, the other classic use is the basis for stuffing. Then there's my mum's trick of serving them mixed in with the sprouts for Christmas dinner. Nice.

## Chestnut, sage and cranberry stuffing

Chicken pieces cooked just plain are usually a bit naff. So rather than reserving stuffing for full-on roast dinners, my idea for this recipe is a really quick, simple stuffing that you actually just tuck under the skin of chicken pieces before roasting them.

### For 4-6 large, skin-on chicken pieces

200 g (7 oz) chestnuts, cooked and peeled
and roughly chopped
50 g (1¾ oz) dried cranberries, finely chopped
4 shallots, finely diced
8 fresh sage leaves, finely chopped
1 tbsp extra virgin olive oil
Sea salt and black pepper

Combine all the ingredients in a bowl and get to work with a potato masher. Pretty quick you'll have a rough, coarse stuffing mixture ■ Pack the mixture together, then divide equally according to the numbers of chicken pieces you have ■ Carefully push the mixture under the skin of the chicken pieces, making sure it is distributed evenly, then simply roast as normal.

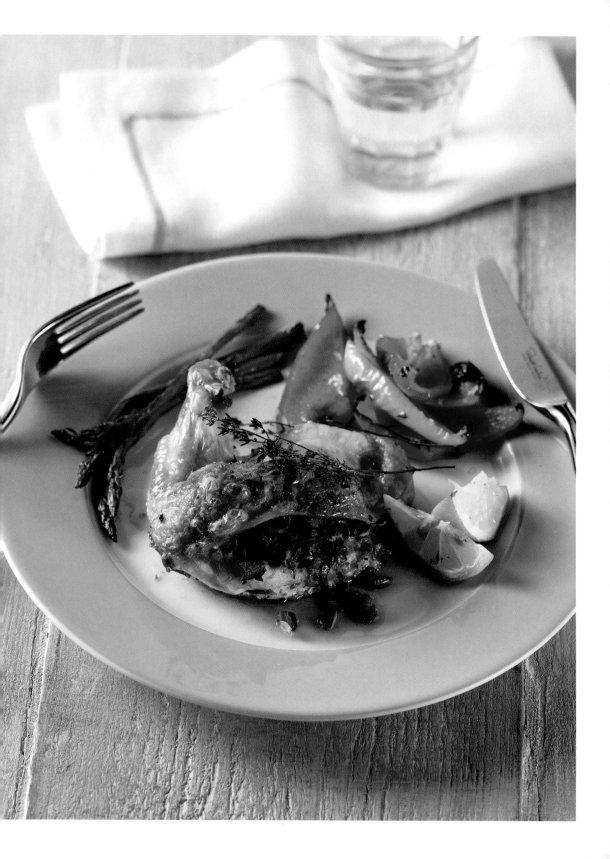

# Spinach

We have Popeye to thank for giving spinach its iconic health status, and for good reason, too.

## Why you should be eating it

Just like Popeye's biceps, spinach is bulging with goodness, jam-packed with carotenoids, vitamin C, folate, vitamin K and magnesium.

Vitamin K is worth a heads-up here, with increasing interest in its important role in keeping bones strong and healthy. Bones need more than just calcium alone, and vitamin K, found aplenty in the dark green leafy stuff, is a key player.

Spinach, like other green leafy veggies, is rich in carotenoids, a family of highly coloured pigments found in plants. As well as brimming with beta carotene, spinach also contains oodles of two other carotenoids, lutein and zeaxanthin. And a diet containing plenty of these two fellas may help to keep eyes healthy as we age, potentially reducing the risk of age-related macular degeneration and cataracts.

When it comes to its antioxidant properties, spinach, just like Popeye, punches above its weight. Amongst other things, there's increasing interest in how some of the clever compounds found in colourful fruits and vegetables might help to protect brain function from deteriorating with age. It seems to work okay for rats anyway, although quite how that translates to us humans remains to be seen.

## How to buy it

The fresher the better, with lush deep green leaves and no signs of wilting.

## How to cook it

Baby spinach works great in salads. Otherwise, spinach can be steamed, sautéed, added to soups, or my fave, added to a stompingly good home-made curry.

# Smoked salmon with spinach and poached egg on rye

Okay, so this probably won't be happening on a work day. But come the weekend, there can't be many better things to roll out of bed for than this.

### Serves 2

4 handfuls of spinach, washed and trimmed of any really thick stalks
1 tbsp of malt vinegar
4 eggs
4 slices of rye or wholemeal (whole-wheat) bread
Small knob of butter
Black pepper
4 sheets of smoked salmon

Take a large-ish frying pan, toss in the washed spinach and put on a low heat. You won't need to add any water as the leaves will wilt and cook of their own accord. They should take about 5 minutes or so ■ Now take a saucepan, half fill with water and bring it to the boil. Add a tablespoon of ordinary malt vinegar and turn down to a really low simmer. Crack the eggs and drop them gently into the pan. You want them to poach as slowly as possible ■ Put the bread in the toaster ■ Go back to the spinach, add the knob of butter and season with black pepper. Give it a good stir ■ Lightly butter the toast. Lay two pieces of salmon across each one. Top with the spinach ■ Now return to the eggs and switch off the heat. Taking a slotted spoon carefully remove them one at a time, shaking off any excess water ■ Place them on top of the spinach and finish off with another smattering of black pepper.

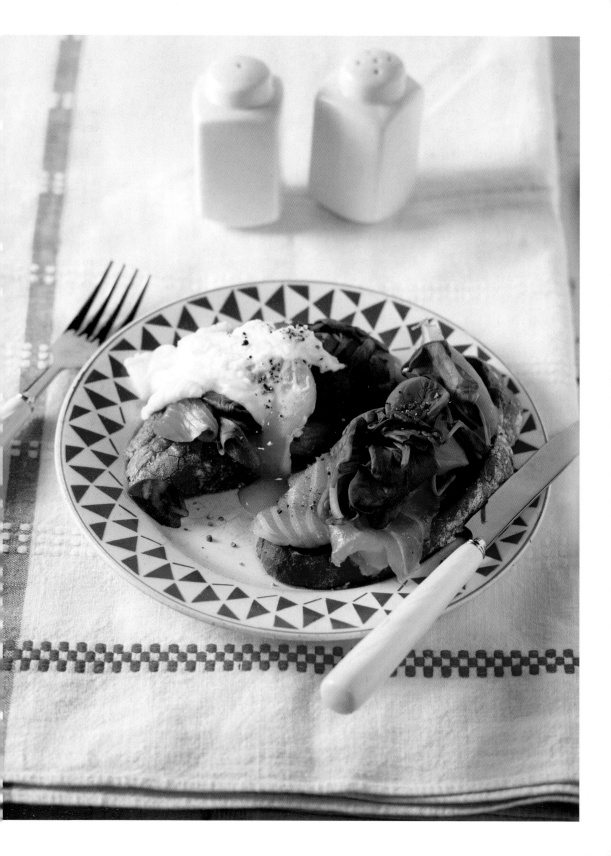

# 9 Kids

The nutritional quality of the food we feed our kids is really important, but it's just as important that they enjoy their food and tuck in. As far as I'm concerned we've got far too many youngsters growing up with a bad relationship with food. On the one hand eating too much junk and getting fat, on the other, starvation diets to be as thin as possible. Either way, that's bad news for the future health of our children.

It might be easier said than done, but helping youngsters to develop a positive relationship with food is likely to stand them in good stead for later in life. In my experience, one of the best ways to do that is to get them more hands-on when it comes to preparing food in the kitchen. Inevitably that means there'll probably be a bit more mess to clear up at the end, but it's a small price to pay if it gets them enthusiastic about food and gives them the skills and knowledge that will see them right when the time comes for them to fend for themselves.

The recipes in this chapter are designed for older, school-age kids, rather than for babies, toddlers or younger pre-school children, as some of the ingredients such as honey (not suitable until a year old), or too much in the way of wholegrain cereals (proportionally too high in fibre), aren't suitable until the little ones get a bit older.

# Turkey

I'm not at all up for feeding my son Olly, or any child for that matter, mechanically recovered poultry that has been squashed into playful shapes. That's just wrong. To be honest, I'd think twice about feeding that stuff to my dear old cat Jasper, and I bet even he'd turn his nose up.

### Why you should be eating it

First up, turkey is a great source of protein, especially useful for rapidly growing kids. But the bonus here is that it provides all that great protein without the higher levels of saturated fats that you might find in some cuts of red meat and processed meat products. Having said that modern methods of feeding poultry high energy diets for rapid weight gain might mean that they're fattier than they may traditionally have been.

Along with its high-quality protein, turkey also supplies good levels of the often hard to get enough of selenium, accompanied by useful amounts of zinc, crucial for normal growth and development, along with vitamin B3, important for making energy from our food, and vitamin B6, needed for the functioning of the nervous system and making brain chemicals that help regulate mood.

### How to buy it

Free-range or organic is preferable. You know the score.

### How to cook it

Whilst a traditional roast turkey is great, remember that you can buy turkey pieces or even mince, which makes for a great alternative in spag bol, burgers or a chilli.

## Turkey burgers

I'm up for just about anything that involves feeding kids proper, healthy food rather than the processed and heavily-marketed stuff, and these burgers will go down a treat.

### Serves 4

450 g (1 lb) free range turkey mince (ground turkey)
2 garlic cloves, crushed
2 tbsp fresh parsley, finely chopped
2 shallots, finely chopped
2 tsp Dijon mustard
2 egg yolks
70 g (3 oz) wholemeal (whole-wheat) breadcrumbs (2 slices of bread)
Black pepper

TO SERVE
4 wholemeal (whole-wheat) rolls, halved
Grated Cheddar cheese
Mayonnaise
Lettuce, finely shredded
Sliced tomato

Mix all the burger ingredients together, mixing well with your hands. Divide the mixture into four and make into burgers about 1.5 cm (¾ in) thick (if they seem too big for small mouths, then it's fine to vary the size and make smaller ones) ■ Grill under a preheated grill until thoroughly cooked through, approximately 10 minutes each side ■ When cooked, put each burger onto the bottom half of the rolls and cover with grated cheese. Place back under the grill to melt the cheese. Spread the top half of the roll with a thin spread of mayo ■ To serve, top the burger with the lettuce and tomato and crown with the top half of the roll.

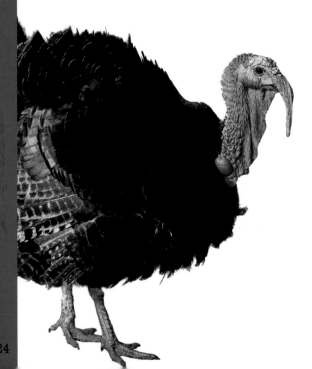

# Sweet potato

I'm a massive fan of sweet potatoes. In my house they're just as much a staple, if not more so, than the more traditional white potatoes.

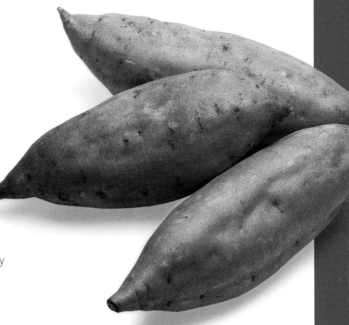

## Why you should be eating it

Whilst we tend to think that vitamin C only comes from fruit such as oranges or kiwis, the fact is that it's widely available from vegetables, too, and just one medium size sweet potato sets a child or an adult for that matter, well on their way to meeting the daily requirement of this vitamin.

Amongst its many important roles, vitamin C spells good news for the skin. As well as an antioxidant, preventing the damaging effects of free radicals, vitamin C is important for making collagen, which we need to give skin strength and elasticity. Perhaps no surprise then that research has uncovered an association between higher dietary vitamin C intakes and a less wrinkly appearance. So, even if it's just for vanity's sake, there's another reason to tuck into more fruit and veg. And one that just might hold sway if you've got image conscious teenagers to feed.

Sweet potatoes are on par with foods like carrots when it comes to providing a hefty dose of carotenoids, notably beta carotene. Not only can the body use beta carotene to make vitamin A, it's also an antioxidant in its own right. And diets high in beta carotene (from fruits and vegetables, not supplements) have consistently shown protection against chronic diseases such as heart disease and cancer.

## How to buy it

Just like you would with white potatoes, look for sweet potatoes that have no signs of spoilage.

## How to cook it

People are often at a loss with what to do with a sweet potato. But really you can do pretty much what you'd do with the more traditional white potato. Steam, boil, mash, roast or bake. Simple.

## Sweet potato chips

Even kids who turn their noses up at anything resembling a vegetable will be more than happy to tuck into these.

### Serves 4

4 medium sweet potatoes, peeled
1 tbsp olive oil
Sea salt and black pepper

Pre-heat the oven to 190°C/375°F/gas mark 5 ▣ Slice the sweet potatoes longways into wedges just a little bit bigger than a finger ▣ Coat the wedges evenly with olive oil ▣ Add a small amount of sea salt and plenty of black pepper ▣ Place on a baking tray and bake for 45 minutes, turning occasionally to prevent them from sticking and to check they don't burn ▣ Serve as an accompaniment to a main meal in place of potatoes. Turkey Burgers (page 124) or Grilled White Fish with Coriander Pesto (page 106) would both work well. They'd also make a good combo with the Mushy Pesto Peas (page 44) and I reckon a dip would go down a treat. Try my home-made Guacamole (page 108) or a simple yoghurt, lemon and parsley dip. Failing that, a good dollop of tomato ketchup is pretty foolproof!

# Brown rice

I don't know what it is about brown rice, but it does conjure up images of wholefood vegetarian restaurants and hippy food. Maybe that puts some people off? Personally, I quite like the vibe of those places. And they generally know how to cook brown rice to perfection.

## Why you should be eating it

Regularly consuming wholegrains, such as brown rice gets a big thumbs-up, spelling good news when it comes to reducing the risk of such serious health problems as heart disease, diabetes and some cancers. That's likely down to the decent levels of fibre, along with the whole kit and caboodle of B-vitamins, minerals and numerous beneficial plant compounds crammed into the wholegrain package.

And generally speaking, the brown stuff is a whole lot better for you than the refined white stuff, which is stripped of a lot of those nutritional goodies. Of course, rice is also naturally gluten-free making it a boon for anyone needing to adhere to a gluten-free diet.

It's worth bearing in mind that whilst high-fibre foods like brown rice are good for older children and adults, younger children need proportionally less fibre. Pre-school children need plenty of energy from their food to grow and develop but only have small stomachs, so whilst it's important to encourage a healthy, varied diet, a low-fat and high-fibre diet may mean they don't get enough energy or nutrients to thrive.

## How to buy it

For a bit of extra flavour, rather than the common-or-garden brown rice, check out brown basmati instead.

## How to cook it

There is a trick to cooking brown rice perfectly. The important bit to get right is to use twice the amount of water to rice. So for every 1 cup of rice, you need 2 cups of water. Bring to the boil, cover and simmer, and the rice is cooked to perfection when all the water has gone.

# Basmati rice frittata

Making good use of basic storecupboard ingredients, this take on frittata shows that it's possible to eat in style without breaking the bank. It also makes veggies a bit less scary for the kids. For this recipe I recommend cooking the rice from scratch and using it straight away in the frittata. That's because storing and re-heating cooked rice can lead to food poisoning (especially if cooked rice is left hanging around at room temperature for too long). And no one needs that.

### Serves 4

150 g (5 oz) brown basmati rice
25 g (1 oz) unsalted butter
1 red (bell) pepper, diced
1 x 200 g (7 oz) tin sweetcorn (corn), no salt or sugar added
5 free range eggs
50 g (2 oz) Parmesan, grated
Black pepper
Good handful of parsley, chopped

Bring the rice to the boil in double the quantity of water, cover and simmer until cooked. It's cooked when it's tender and all the water has been absorbed ▧ Melt the butter in a non-stick frying pan (about 25 cm/10 in in diameter). Gently fry the diced red pepper until soft, add the sweetcorn and just-cooked rice and heat through ▧ Break the eggs into a bowl and beat them well. Add the grated cheese, a good dash of black pepper, parsley and mix well. Add the cooked pepper, sweetcorn and rice to the egg mix and stir through. Pour it all back into the frying pan ▧ Turn the heat down to very low and cook the frittata until it is set on the bottom and just runny on the top, about 15 minutes. Preheat the grill to its highest setting and flash the pan underneath to finish ▧ To serve, cut into 4 wedges, loosen all around the edges with a palette knife and slide gently onto plates.

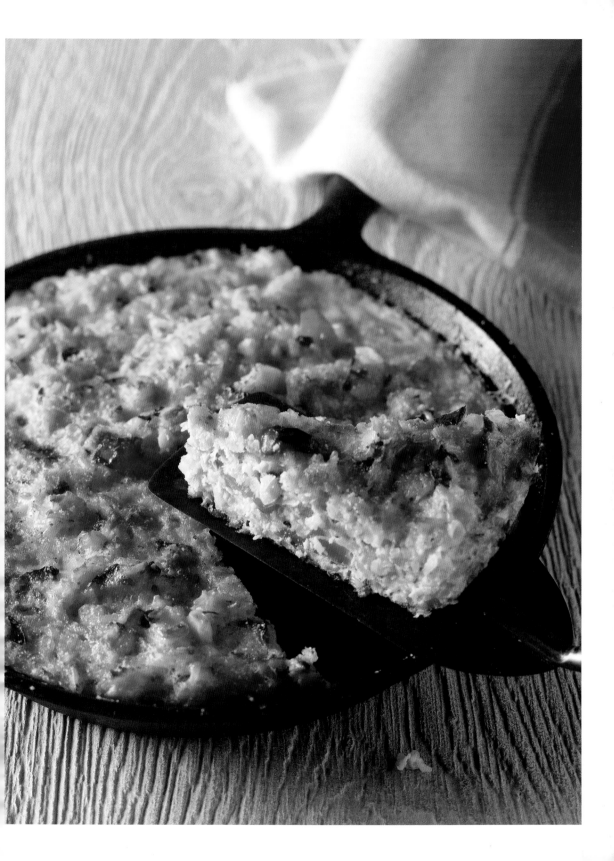

# Wholewheat

It seems like every other person has a food intolerance to wheat these days. And I have to admit that I do frequently come across people who feel better for cutting down their intake. Maybe we just eat too much of the stuff? But I'm not one of the anti-wheat brigade. If you're not allergic or intolerant to it, it's got a lot of good points in its wholegrain form.

## Why you should be eating it

We've all heard the marketing jive about wholegrain goodness. In all fairness, they've got it pretty much bang on (for once!). Consuming wholegrains, such as wholewheat, appears to impart plenty of health benefits. Population-based studies show an association between consumption of wholegrains and a reduced risk of heart disease, some cancers, diabetes and to plonk a cherry on top, obesity.

This who's who of health benefits can be explained in part by the generous dose of dietary fibre served up by wholegrains. But there's a whole lot more to grains such as wholewheat than just fibre, containing useful amounts of B-vitamins, various minerals, and like other plant foods, a dazzling array of beneficial phytochemicals. So if your penchant is for the refined white stuff, you might want to get with the whole (grain) package.

It's worth remembering that whilst high fibre foods like wholewheat are good for older children and adults, younger children need proportionally less fibre in their diets. See Brown Rice on page 126 for more on this.

## How to buy it

The potential health benefits of wheat are realized from having it in its unadulterated wholegrain form. That means opting for wholemeal bread, wholewheat pasta, wholemeal flour and whole-wheat flakes.

## How to cook it

They say don't teach your granny to suck eggs, but here goes anyway. Sandwiches, pasta, home-made pizza, wholegrain breakfast cereals and muesli. Enough said.

## Pitta pizza

Most kids love pizza and this simplified version feeds hungry mouths in minutes. Cold, it also makes a great addition to the lunch box.

PER CHILD
1 wholemeal (whole-wheat) pitta bread
1 tbsp tomato purée (tomato paste)
1 tsp extra virgin olive oil
A good pinch of dried mixed herbs

FOR THE TOPPING
¼ green (bell) pepper, finely diced
1 thinly sliced mushroom
1 tbsp sweetcorn (corn)
½ tin sardines, drained and cut in half longways
Grated Cheddar cheese

Divide the pitta bread into two separate halves and lightly toast on both sides (but if you like a thicker pizza base, just leave the pitta whole, which works just fine, too) ■ Mix together the tomato purée, olive oil and mixed herbs ■ Spread the tomato paste over the inside of each pitta ■ Add any combination of toppings ■ Grill under a medium heat until the pitta pizza is piping hot.

# Buckwheat

I'm all for introducing a bit more diversity into people's diets and eating a variety of wholegrains, rather than just wheat and wheat-based products, is one way of doing that. And before you think I've gone and lost the plot, despite its name, buckwheat is completely unrelated to wheat as we know it.

### Why you should be eating it

Whilst not technically a grain, its culinary use is as such. And there's no reason to think that the benefits associated with wholegrain consumption don't apply, namely an association with a reduced risk of chronic health problems, such as heart disease, some cancers, diabetes and obesity.

That's likely to be in part to do with buckwheat's high fibre credentials, but it's also a plentiful source of magnesium. As well as being needed for things like healthy bones and muscle function, magnesium also helps us turn our food into energy. Buckwheat also provides complex carbohydrates, along with a good range of B-vitamins also involved in energy production, meaning that this is a good fuel to put in the tank.

Do keep in mind that buckwheat is a high-fibre food and whilst wholegrains such as this are great for older children and adults, younger children need proportionally less fibre in their diets. See Brown Rice on page 126 for more on this.

### How to buy it

Buckwheat comes in various guises. You can buy it either unroasted or a roasted version called Kasha, which has a nuttier flavour. Then there are flakes, flour and not forgetting noodles, too.

### How to cook it

Buckwheat can be used in place of rice as a side dish, the flour is great for pancakes, the flakes for porridge or muesli and the noodles a perfect accompaniment to a stir-fry.

## Lemon and raisin buckwheat pancakes

This is bound to get the young ones queuing up for more and probably the adults, too.

**Makes 12-15 pancakes**

100 g (3½ oz) buckwheat flour
100 g (3½ oz) wholemeal plain (whole-wheat all-purpose) flour
2 tsp baking powder
2 free range eggs, lightly beaten
1 tbsp extra virgin olive oil
25 ml (9 fl oz) semi-skimmed (2% milkfat) milk
3 tbsp honey
3 tbsp lemon juice
100 g (3½ oz) raisins
Groundnut oil (or olive oil in cases of peanut allergy)

Sift the flours and baking powder into a large mixing bowl, rubbing out all the lumps. Tip in the bran left from the wholemeal flour ■ Make a well in the centre of the flour and tip in the eggs, olive oil and milk and whisk until blended and smooth. Whisk in the honey and lemon juice. Finally stir in the raisins ■ Leave to stand for 30 minutes ■ Heat a teaspoon of groundnut/olive oil in a non-stick frying pan and drop in a dessert spoon of the mixture. Spread it around so you get a small pancake of roughly 10 cm (4 in) in diameter. Depending on the size of your pan, you can cook a couple of them at a time. Leave the pancakes to cook until they look dry on top with little holes appearing, turn and cook for a further few minutes on the other side ■ Serve straight away or cool and leave for later when you can simply grill them ■ Serve just on their own or with sliced banana and a drizzle of honey or maple syrup.

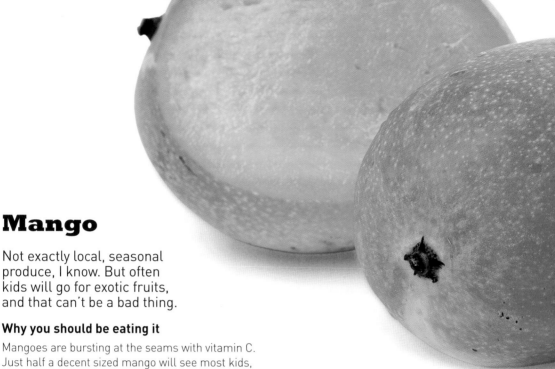

# Mango

Not exactly local, seasonal produce, I know. But often kids will go for exotic fruits, and that can't be a bad thing.

### Why you should be eating it

Mangoes are bursting at the seams with vitamin C. Just half a decent sized mango will see most kids, not to mention adults, well on their way to getting their daily requirement. Good stuff.

Then there's plenty of beta carotene, too. Getting plenty of this antioxidant from the diet (but not from supplements) is linked with a reduced risk of heart disease and cancer. And as it happens, beta carotene from fruits such as mango appears to be more efficiently absorbed than from veggies such as the green leafies. Perhaps that goes some way to overcoming the perennial problem of getting kids to eat their greens!

And just to tip my hat once more to the rich diversity of naturally occurring compounds in fruit and veg, there's a sniff of interest in a plant compound called lupeol. This is found in a range of fruits, including mango, and researchers are beginning to look at its potential role as an anti-cancer agent. Whilst that in itself is not reason enough to eat mangoes, it does go to show what an amazing array of beneficial compounds we're likely to take on board by eating a good mix of fruit and veg.

### How to buy it

Steer clear of the bullet-hard unripe mangoes that crop up far too often in supermarkets. Instead keep your eyes peeled for the semi-soft ripe ones ready for feasting on.

### How to cook it

Pretty much a case of eat as-is. Mango is great chopped up and added to breakfast cereal or fruit salads or blitzed in a smoothie.

## Frozen mango smoothie

This should go down as welcome refreshment for kids running riot on hot sunny days.

### Serves 2

1 ripe mango
200 ml (7 fl oz) fresh orange juice
1 tbsp honey
8 ice cubes

This requires some planning ahead as you need to freeze the mango in advance. To do this, peel the mango and slice the flesh into chunks. Place on a tray and freeze ▓ When you're ready to make the smoothie, place the frozen mango chunks, orange juice, honey and ice cubes in a blender and blend until smooth ▓ If it's too thick and difficult to blend, just add a touch more orange juice to get it going. You're basically looking for a thick, fruity, icy slush.

# Blueberries

Blueberries are often hailed as the daddy of all superfoods. The problem with that is the concept of the 'superfood' is a load of ridiculous drivel. Whilst the marketing execs might be wed to this concept, it's time we, the consumer, filed for divorce and instead got hitched to the idea that it's whole diets – not single foods – that reap the real benefits in the long run.

### Why you should be eating it

Don't get me wrong, I'm not bashing blueberries. Their potential health benefits are pretty impressive. They are an insanely good source of antioxidants, trouncing virtually every other fruit and veg going. But my guess is that you probably know that already.

Here's the drill. Blueberries are awash with a wide diversity of naturally occurring phytochemicals. Or in everyday talk, a whole bunch of useful stuff that plants make. Chief amongst these are the anthocyanins, plant pigments responsible for the blueberry's radiant blue-purple colouring.

All of this has sparked interest in the way berry phytochemicals might improve our health, for example, as possible protective dietary factors against the development of cancer or cardiovascular disease. Blueberries in particular may also have a role to play in preventing age-related declines in brain function, possibly through antioxidant effects, anti-inflammatory effects or indeed a number of other mechanisms. Feeding them to aged rats seems to do the trick anyway. But only time will tell if us humans can expect to derive the same benefits.

### How to buy it

They're at their best fresh but that's not always possible or affordable, so I wouldn't hesitate to opt for frozen blueberries as a fall back.

### How to cook it

Just like other berries, they're great to snack on, added to summer fruit salads or yoghurt, generously scattered on to muesli or porridge or given the blender treatment for smoothies.

## Blueberry lollies

Sometimes kids don't like a food because of the way it looks, especially if it looks remotely healthy. But it's all about the packaging. Make it look like a lolly and you're laughing.

### Makes 4 x 100ml lollies

125 g (4½ oz) blueberries, fresh or defrosted
100 ml (4 fl oz) natural yoghurt
1 banana

Whizz everything in the blender and pour into lolly moulds ▦ Place in the freezer. After an hour, give them a good stir with the stick scraping round the sides to break up any ice crystals ▦ Freeze for a further hour and you've got yourself a healthy treat for the little ones (and most probably the grown-ups, too).

**KIDS**

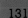

131

# 10 Desserts

Bring it on! I love desserts but I try not to have them too often. It's nothing to do with worrying about my waistline or anything like that, I just don't always have enough time to make them the way I like them, and that's homemade. Personally, I'd rather go without than have a pre-packaged job, which could be loaded with sugar and laced with additives. That's just not my style. When it comes to desserts, I apply pretty much the same criteria as I would to other food. It's got to taste good but also do me some good.

What would a chapter on desserts be without chocolate? Dark chocolate features regularly in my diet. It's probably the one single food I would miss more than any other if I couldn't have it. And there's a good reason that it's made it into my top 100 list. Scientific research is beginning to show that chocolate (well, the cocoa bit) has more in common with a health food than a junk food.

Where possible I've tried to make use of ingredients that add some nutritional value to the diet without adding masses of sugar. But I won't pretend they're all ultra-healthy either. They're not. But, come on, who wants to be good all the time anyway? That's got to be too much like hard work.

But best of all, I've pinched a couple of my mum's recipes. Good times!

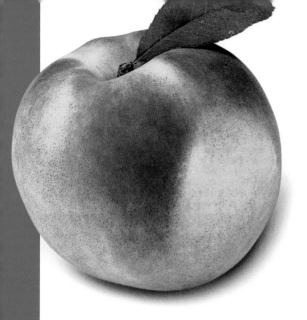

## How to cook it

Bought ripe and in-season, there's no better way than eating them just as they are. They're also great sliced into muesli or porridge or added to smoothies. Peaches can also be cooked, being an integral part of some classic dessert dishes such as peach melba.

## Peaches with honey-vanilla wine

Most days I'd never have time for this, but when I've got friends over for food, and I want to pull a blinder out the bag, this is the one.

Serves 4

2 tsp ground arrowroot
200 ml (7 fl oz) white wine, at room temperature
2 tbsp honey
1 vanilla pod
4 ripe peaches at room temperate

Mix the ground arrowroot with a few spoonfuls of the white wine and stir until it's blended and smooth ■ Gently warm the rest of the wine and honey. Split the vanilla pod along its length and scrape out the tiny black seeds with a teaspoon. Add the seeds to the honey and wine, and give it a little whisk to distribute the seeds evenly. Add the blended arrowroot and warm through, stirring constantly until it thickens. Do not bring it to the boil as it will turn cloudy and spoil. As soon as the sauce has thickened, remove the pan from the heat ■ When ready to serve prepare the peaches. Lightly score each fruit, following the natural line marking the sides of the stone with the tip of a knife. Immerse the fruit in a bowl of boiling water for a few moments. Take them out with a spoon and carefully peel away the skins, if you haven't got cooks' fingers you may need plastic gloves for this. Then run a knife round the fruit again, this time going down to the stone and gently break them in half. Remove the stone and place each half upright in a grillproof serving dish ■ Pour over the warm sauce and grill for 5-7 minutes until the peaches are just brown and bubbling ■ Serve with a little sauce spooned in the stone hole, and some crème fraîche or natural yoghurt on the side.

# Peaches

Whilst never likely to be branded a superfood (and a good job, too), peaches are a reliable all-rounder, can bump up our daily intake of fresh fruit and veg and provide much needed variety to the average diet.

### Why you should be eating it

Peaches are rich in antioxidants, including the usual suspects such as vitamin C, along with a smidgen of carotenoids. Add in a good measure of dietary fibre, some potassium, a sprinkling of other vitamins and minerals, and myriad beneficial plant compounds, and we have a pretty healthy concoction.

Let's be clear about one thing. On the whole, most people just don't eat enough fruit and vegetables. A minimum of 5-a-day fruit and veg offers significant health benefits, and 6, 7 or 8-a-day probably even more. It's a pretty smart health insurance policy with good evidence that a diet containing plenty of fruits and veggies reduces the risk of chronic diseases, such as heart disease, stroke and cancer. And that's why peaches get the thumbs up.

### How to buy it

Buy them ripe by checking that the fruit is semi-soft, but give any that have gone squidgy a wide berth.

# Strawberries

Strawberries symbolize summertime and picnics and are a great example of fantastic home-grown produce.

## Why you should be eating it

Strawberries are a ridiculously good source of vitamin C, one of the roles of which is to function as an antioxidant, protecting the body from the damaging effects of free radicals. All in all that fits with the strawberry's reputation as an antioxidant heavyweight.

Strawberries offer up a veritable bounty of beneficial plant compounds. Notable amongst these are a class of flavonoids known as anthocyanins, the plant pigments responsible for the vivid hue of berries.

Whilst these are considered important contributors to the total antioxidant properties of the fruit, absorption of these compounds is pretty poor to say the least and what is absorbed is excreted rapidly. So when push comes to shove, that basically means it's unlikely that enough of these compounds get in to the body to have a really meaningful antioxidant effect, and most likely they exert their beneficial effects through other mechanisms. In particular, researchers are interested in the potential of these plant compounds to keep the brain and our cognitive faculties healthy as we age, along with possible benefits for cardiovascular health, even cancer-prevention, although it's early days and there's simply a lack of research in humans to be certain about any of this. Like you really needed any more encouragement to tuck in!

## How to buy it

There's nothing more disappointing than insipid-tasting, rubbery strawberries bought out of season. I feel totally gutted when I eat those because I know they should be tasting at least 100 times better. So keep it real and make the most of freshly picked fruits from local farms when they're bang in season. Best of all, brave the great outdoors for a spot of Pick-Your-Own.

## How to cook it

Really fresh, fully ripened, peak season strawberries are pretty blissful just as they are. They also make a great addition to fruit salads, chopped up in muesli or porridge, or blitzed into a smoothie.

## Strawberries with basil and lemon

I know I keep banging on about seasonal food, and you've got to trust me on this one. No messing around, you need properly ripe, super-sweet, bang-in-season strawberries for this little number.

**Serves 4**

500 g (1 lb) ripe strawberries, topped
    and halved lengthways
2 tbsp finely shredded fresh basil leaves
Zest of 1 and juice of ½ an unwaxed lemon
Crème fraîche or Greek yoghurt, to serve

Remove the stalks of each strawberry and slice in half, lengthways. Place them into a serving bowl and sprinkle over the shredded basil, lemon zest and juice. If you took no notice of my advice and the strawberries aren't that sweet, use a little less lemon juice ■ Toss very, very gently to combine the flavours and leave for at least half an hour before serving ■ Serve with crème fraîche or Greek yoghurt.

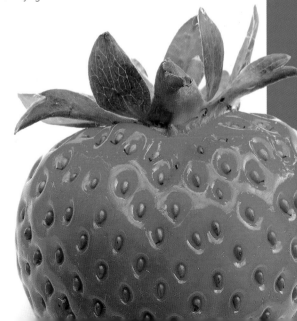

# Dark (Semisweet) chocolate

Right from when I was a kid I knew that Willy Wonka was on to something.

## Why you should be eating it

Cocoa contains an array of bio-active compounds. These include large amounts of naturally occurring phytochemicals, notably a subclass of flavonoids called flavanols.

Evidence is accumulating that regular consumption of dark chocolate may hold benefits for cardiovascular health. It does this through various mechanisms. For example, the antioxidants in chocolate may help to protect LDL cholesterol from oxidation, which makes it less likely to clog up artery walls. Another is the effect of cocoa flavanols on making the blood less sticky, helping to prevent blood clots. These clever compounds also appear to help reduce elevated blood pressure, along with improving something called endothelial function, which is important for keeping arteries healthy and working well.

Undoubtedly more research needs to be done to better understand the full health benefits of chocolate and its beneficial plant compounds. And a word of warning – chocolate is a high calorie, energy-dense food, so moderation is the order of the day. And remember what happened to Augustus Gloop...

## How to buy it

To derive the health benefits, maximize the cocoa solids and minimize the added sugar. We're talking dark chocolate here, at least 70 per cent cocoa solids, and watch out for new products that will soon come on to the market that have guaranteed levels of cocoa flavanols. Due to careful processing, these will have significantly higher levels of the beneficial compounds that are typically lost in the manufacture of more run-of-the-mill chocolate.

## How to cook it

Whether eaten on its own, used in desserts or even added to a chilli (see page 43), dark chocolate is one of life's pleasures, so enjoy it to the max.

# Ginger choc-pots

It's no surprise that the chocolate recipe in this book was masterminded by a woman, and that would be Louise, my better half. She cleverly uses a sugar replacement called xylitol for this, which has a lower GI than sugar and actually appears to help prevent tooth decay. You can get it in most supermarkets and health food shops.

### Serves 6

350 g (12½ oz) dark (semisweet) chocolate (70% cocoa solids)
50 g (2 oz) unsalted butter at room temperature
100 g (3½ oz) xylitol
1 tsp vanilla extract
4 large eggs
50 g (2 oz) brown rice or quinoa flour
2½ cm (1 in) chunk fresh root ginger, peeled and finely grated

Pre-heat the oven to 200°C/400°F/gas mark 6 ▨ Lightly butter 6 small ovenproof pots and line with baking paper ▨ Break the chocolate into rough pieces and melt in a bain marie over a pan of simmering water. Allow to cool to room temperature ▨ Blend the butter with the xylitol to form a smooth consistency. Add the vanilla extract, eggs and flour and mix ▨ Stir the chocolate into the mixture and add the grated ginger, pour into the buttered pots ▨ Place the pots onto a baking tray and cook in the oven for 10-12 minutes.

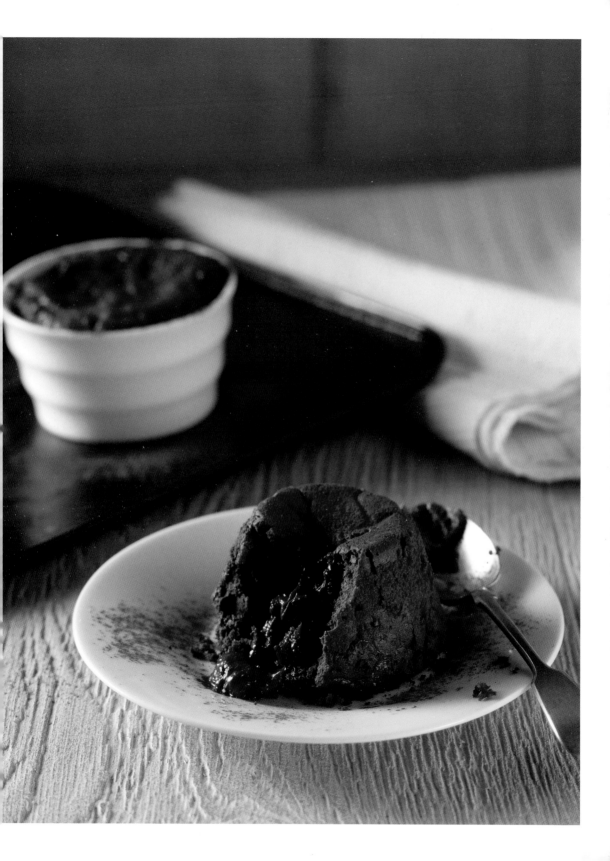

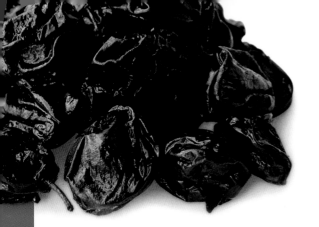

## How to cook it

You'll probably get zilch by way of foodie street cred for this, but I reckon prunes make for a great snack just as they are. Rehydrated or partially rehydrated ones are the best for this. Prunes are also great added to porridge or muesli, fruit salads, desserts and even savoury dishes, such as roast pork or in place of apricots in a tagine.

# Prunes

I've been thinking about it now for a whole 5 minutes and I can't think of a single food that is more uncool than the prune. But prunes can have a certain charm and are just as good as any of those heavily marketed superfoods.

### Why you should be eating it

Appearance aside, I suspect one of the reasons that prunes are perceived as being a bit unglamorous is their reputation as a cure for constipation. And we shouldn't really hold that against them, as I don't imagine many other laxatives taste quite as nice as they do. The 'regularity' effect is most likely due to the high fibre nature of prunes, along with high levels of a type of sugar called sorbitol.

Boasting a high level of phenolic compounds, prunes are also jammed full of health-promoting antioxidants. In fact, compared with other fruits and veg, they're up there with the big boys. They're also a great source of boron, which combined with a decent bit of vitamin K, offer a nutritional duo to promote bone health. Add to the mix the good levels of potassium found in prunes and we also have a food that is likely to be beneficial for cardiovascular health.

### How to buy it

In the highly unlikely event that you didn't know this already, prunes are dried plums, so typically you would buy them in their dried form. More recently it's possible to get them partially rehydrated, which makes them good to go straight out the packet.

## Slow-cooked dried fruit and white tea compote

This might sound a bit experimental but it tastes fantastic. The one bit of kit you need is a slow-cooker. If you don't own one, they're a real hidden treasure and worth every penny.

2 white tea bags
3 cups boiling water
4 tbsp maple syrup
100 g (4 oz) prunes
50 g (2 oz) dried pineapple, cut into large chunks
50 g (2 oz) dried mango, cut into large chunks
50 g (2 oz) dried apricots, halved
50 g (2 oz) dried apple rings, cut into large chunks
1 unwaxed orange, zest and juice
Zest of 1 unwaxed lemon
1 cinnamon stick, halved
2 star anise
Greek yoghurt, to serve

Steep the white tea bags in boiling water for 3 minutes before removing. Dissolve the maple syrup in the hot tea ■ Add to the slow cooker, along with the dried fruit, orange juice, orange and lemon zest, cinnamon and the star anise. Stir well, cover and cook on low for around 4 hours ■ You'll know it's ready when the fruit is melt-in-the-mouth tender and the liquid has reduced to a syrupy consistency ■ Remove the cinnamon pieces and star anise ■ Remove the compote from the slow cooker and allow to cool. Cover, then refrigerate until chilled ■ Lovely served up with some authentic Greek yoghurt.

# Pineapple

I'm all for making the most of the amazing local, seasonal produce that's out there. But, from time to time, I do get tempted to commit a bit of food mile heresy and indulge in something exotic and tropical.

### Why you should be eating it

A generous slice of pineapple provides abundant vitamin C, and is a big step towards meeting the average daily requirement for this vitamin. Vitamin C is not only an important antioxidant vitamin, protecting the body from the ravages of damaging free radicals, but it's also vital to maintaining healthy connective tissue in the skin, cartilage and bone, due to its role in the production of collagen. Stress and smoking are both factors that can rapidly use up vitamin C.

Of course, we can't just reduce complex foods down to one or two nutrients. Pineapple, like other fruits, contains an array of beneficial plant compounds and it's likely to be the interaction of these, along with the better known nutrients, that account for the substantial health benefits of eating more fruit and veggies.

### How to buy it

At the risk of looking a bit weird in the supermarket, one of the best indicators of ripeness is to pluck one of the green spikes atop the pineapple, and if it dislodges easily, you've bagged a ripe one.

### How to cook it

Freshly sliced pineapple makes for a great summer snack just as it is, and is equally good in smoothies and fruit salads, even salsa. Pineapple also works a treat with savoury dishes such as pork, poultry and seafood.

## Spiced pineapple compote

If you're well organized you can make the syrup for this the day before so that the spices have loads of time to infuse all that lovely flavour.

Serves 4

6 tbsp maple syrup
½ cinnamon stick
1 star anise
1 tbsp dark rum
Zest of ½ an unwaxed lemon
125 ml (4 fl oz) water
1 ripe pineapple, peeled, cored and chopped into chunks

Make up the syrup first. Place all the ingredients, except the pineapple, in a small pan with the water. Bring to the boil and simmer for a few minutes. Take off the heat and allow to cool ■ When you're ready to serve, gently warm the pineapple with the syrup for a few minutes. You don't want to stew the pineapple – just warm it through ■ Remove the cinnamon stick and star anise and serve in glass bowls with crème fraîche or natural yoghurt on the side.

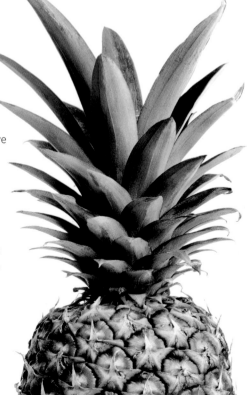

# Pecan nuts

We tend not to consider nuts as healthy foods. Maybe that's because all too often they come smothered in salt or some sort of sugary coating. Or because of our general fat-phobia and mistrust of any food that's not ultra low fat. Time for a re-think.

## Why you should be eating it

Whilst a diet high in saturated fats, found in foods such as fatty or processed meat, full fat dairy products, cakes, biscuits and pastries for example, is implicated in heart disease, the same can't be said for the unsaturated fats that predominate in pecans. Unlike saturated fats, which tend to bump up levels of 'bad' LDL cholesterol levels, the 'good' fats in pecan nuts tends to reduce it. And it looks likely that nuts also contain a whole kit and caboodle of bio-active constituents, everything from cholesterol-lowering plant sterols, to fibre, phenolic compounds, vitamin E, magnesium, and more besides, which collectively bolster their heart-healthy credentials.

But pecans are no one-trick pony. When we think of antioxidants, we don't really associate them with nuts. But pecans ooze antioxidant prowess. And that's important because many chronic diseases, let's say cancer, heart disease, Alzheimer's disease, in fact the ageing process itself, may partly be due to something called oxidative stress. And a diet containing plenty of antioxidant-rich foods may go some way to counteracting that.

And despite all that fat and all those calories, nuts tend to be foods that are satiating. And that may be why regular consumers of nuts, if anything, tend to be slimmer than those who give them a wide berth.

## How to buy it

Looking to purchase your pecans from a shop with a good turnover of stock should help to ensure freshness. And just as importantly, to keep them in tip top nick, they're best stored in an air-tight container in the fridge to prevent their high content of unsaturated fats from going rancid.

## How to cook it

Pecans are great for just snacking, chopped and added to muesli or scattered on to porridge or yoghurt with a drizzle of maple syrup.

# Dark chocolate pecan brownies

This is a corker. It might not be whiter-than-white healthy, but crammed full of dark chocolate and pecans, it's got crazy amounts of antioxidants and beneficial plant compounds, scoring some serious... err... brownie points.

175 g (6 oz) dark (semisweet) chocolate (70% cocoa solids)
125 g (3½ oz) unsalted butter at room temperature
8 tbsp maple syrup
2 large eggs
1 tsp baking powder
100 g (3½ oz) brown rice flour
100 g (3½ oz) pecan nuts, roughly chopped
½ tsp vanilla extract

Grease a square cake tin (roughly 25 cm x 15 cm/ 10 in x 6 in) and line with baking paper ■ Break the chocolate into rough pieces and melt in a bain marie over a pan of simmering water. Allow to cool to room temperature ■ In a mixing bowl, combine the butter and maple syrup until the butter is creamy – don't worry if the maple syrup doesn't totally combine with the butter at this stage – the main thing is getting the butter creamed down. Beat the eggs and add to the mixture ■ Slowly stir in the chocolate and mix until smooth. You don't want to end up with scrambled eggs, so make sure the melted chocolate has cooled down before doing this ■ Add the baking powder to the flour and sift before combining into the mixture ■ Add the pecans and vanilla extract, giving the ingredients a final mix ■ Pour the mixture into the cake tin and bake at 180ºC/350ºF/gas mark 4 for 25 minutes. By this point the brownie mixture should feel firm to the touch ■ Allow to cool before cutting into individual brownie squares.

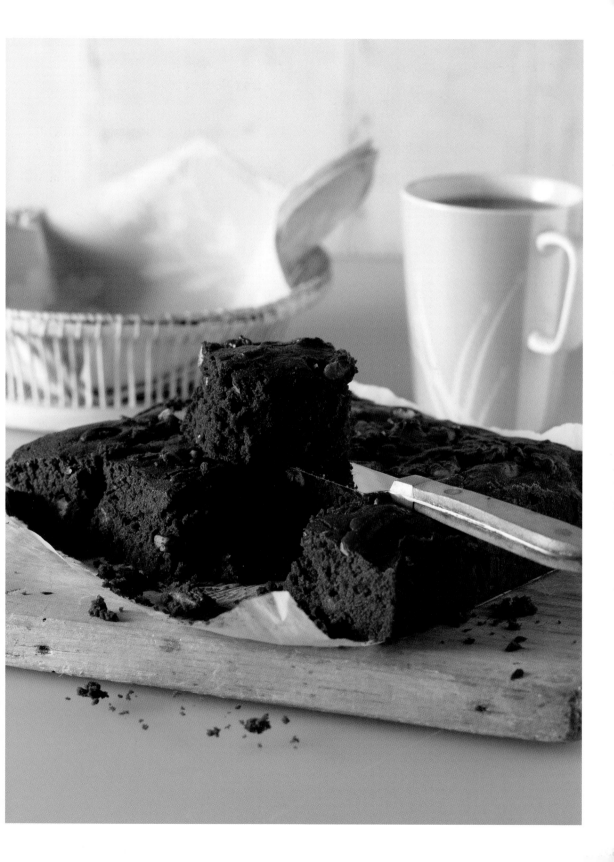

# Drinks

11

Check this out. Tea, coffee and red wine have all made it into my top 100. I'd better come clean and spill the beans by confessing that one of the main reasons they've made it in is because they bring a bit of pleasure to life. After all, isn't that what food and drink are supposed to be all about? Let's face it, life without them just wouldn't be the same. This probably sounds like nutritional heresy, but they've also made it into this book on merit, too. Honest! And that's because there's a decent bit of scientific evidence to show that they confer health benefits. So once and for all, we can kick into touch the idea that anything that tastes remotely good must be bad for us. And about time, too.

That's not to say that tea, coffee and red wine are good for everyone. They aren't. There are certain times (say, pregnancy for example) or certain circumstances, when they're just not appropriate. But where there's no medical or health reason not to indulge in these beverages, in moderation, they've got a lot going for them.

Of course, there's a whole load more to this chapter than a trip to the local coffee shop or bar. A great way to increase intake of fruit is to have it in the form of a drink. And that can really hit the spot on sweltering summer days. I'm also a big fan of getting a bit more in the way of culinary herbs and spices into the diet. Not only are they over-flowing with beneficial plant compounds called phytochemicals, when incorporated into drinks they'll almost always add a bit of funkiness to the proceedings.

So without further ado, it's time for a toast. Here's to your good health. Cheers!

# Watermelon

As its name suggests, watermelon is nearly all water. But the small bit left that isn't water is well worth the effort.

## Why you should be eating it

Anyone would think that tomatoes are the only source of the carotenoid lycopene, the stuff that makes tomatoes red and has been associated with numerous health benefits. Admittedly, tomatoes do account for the majority of our intake, but watermelon is also a meaningful source of this plant pigment and deserves its share of the glory.

Lycopene is a mighty free radical scavenger, and whilst we can't be sure that it will have the same effect when we eat watermelon, consumption of lycopene-rich tomato products has been associated with various health benefits such as reduced incidence of heart disease, some forms of cancer, notably prostate cancer, even protection of the skin against damage from UV light.

And whilst the lycopene from tomatoes is much better absorbed when they've been cooked or processed, it appears that the lycopene from watermelon in its raw state, unlike that of tomatoes, is well absorbed. Bonus.

## How to buy it

Watermelons can be monsters, so if it's something smaller you're after then be on the lookout for shops that will sell them by the half or even by the big fat slice.

And a little tip. If you want to max-up the lycopene, then store whole, intact, watermelons at room temperature, rather than in the fridge. Researchers have shown that synthesis of carotenoids actually continues after harvesting and that this is enhanced by storage at 21°C but inhibited at 5 °C.

## How to cook it

On summer days, watermelon is just perfect by the slice, especially if you stick them in the fridge for a while first. Otherwise, you can scoop out the flesh or cut it into cubes to bring a bit of summertime to any fruit salad.

# Chilled watermelon and lime quencher

This thirst quencher extraordinaire is perfect for a scorcher of a summer day.

Serves 4

½ a medium watermelon
250 ml (9 fl oz) sparkling mineral water, chilled
Juice of 1 lime
2 tbsp clear honey
Slices of lime to serve

Roughly chop the watermelon into chunks, discarding skin and seeds. Place in a bowl and refrigerate for 1 hour ■ When the watermelon has chilled, add it to a blender along with the sparkling water, lime juice and honey. Blend ■ Serve immediately with ice and a slice of lime.

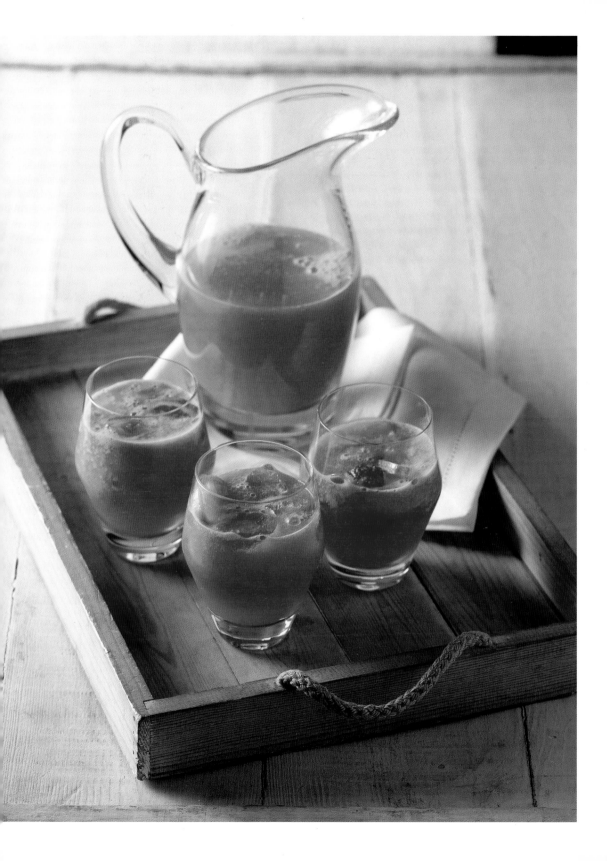

# Pomegranate juice

Flouncing around sipping from a bottle of pomegranate juice (that probably costs almost as much as it does to put food on the table for a family of four) might all be very debonair and quite the mark of the superfood sophisticate. But does pomegranate juice justify the price tag? Read on...

### Why you should be drinking it

Pomegranate juice is a ridiculously good source of antioxidants courtesy of its wealth of polyphenols. The real headline grabbers are the ellagitannins, especially the uniquely abundant punicalagin, but also the likes of anthocyanins and flavonols for good measure. Okay, that's my full quota of big words used up for one day.

What all this stacks up to is a fruit juice that may have some hefty health benefits. First up, pomegranate juice looks to be a strong candidate for a cardio-protective beverage, with some evidence that its heart-friendly plant compounds may help to hinder the build up of fatty deposits in the walls of the arteries (known as atherosclerosis) and subsequently heart disease.

There's also some tantalizing research emerging on the potential anti-cancer properties of pomegranate polyphenols, much of which has focused on prostate cancer. Whilst the data is very preliminary, there is some evidence to indicate that pomegranate juice may offer a helping hand to combat the progression of the disease. Potentially exciting stuff, although loads more research needs to be done before we get too carried away.

### How to buy it

With the inevitable hyperbole that goes with these things, it's no surprise that pomegranate juices are now widely available. But for the quality ones, with a high percentage of pomegranate juice in them, your pocket will take a hit. And beware the pretender pomegranate juice drinks that are full of added sugar or have had little more than a brief encounter with a pomegranate.

### How to cook it

You can take it neat but it also makes for a lavish addition to a home-made smoothie or cocktail.

## Pim-pom cocktail

Whilst I'm not advocating irresponsible drinking (except for when I accidentally do it by mistake), this is quite a party-pleaser. And it works almost as well without the booze for a teetotal version.

FOR ONE GLASS
**One measure of Pimms**
**A third of a glass of orange juice**
**A third of a glass of pomegranate juice**
**Couple of fresh mint leaves**
**Ice**

Measuring out juices and spirits for cocktails is a bit of a fuss, so here it's worked out according to the highly scientific method of how big or small your glass is. Highly technical I know ■ Pour the Pimms and juices into your glass. Stir. Slightly crush the mint leaves so they releases some of their oils and pop those along with the ice into your glass. Then it's straight back to the party.

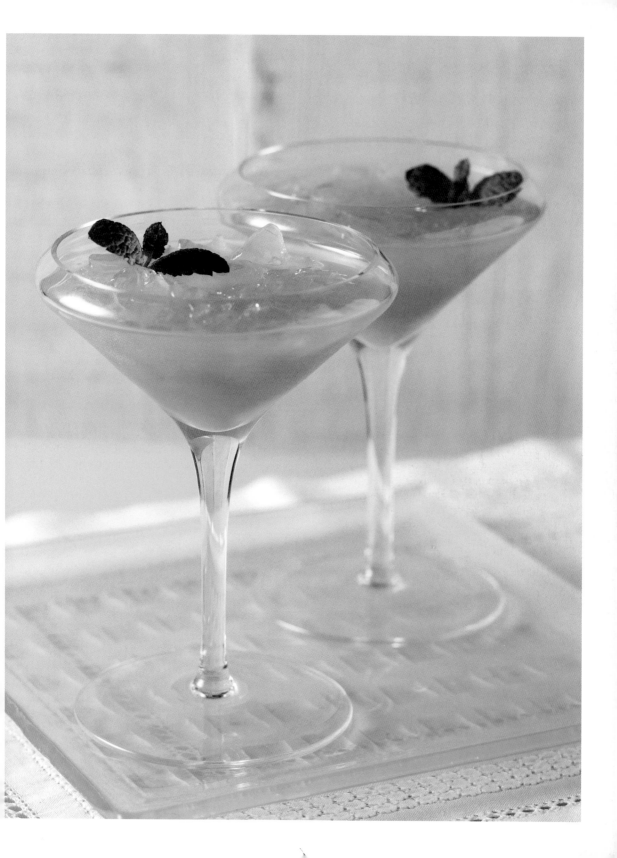

# Mint

Mint isn't just something that comes in toothpaste and chewing gum. The fresh stuff can be used for all sorts of culinary purposes and is just about guaranteed to add a refreshingly cool zing. It may even help keep your digestion in mint condition, too.

## Why you should be eating it

Mint is actually a group of about 25 or so species with a whole lot of different varieties. The most well-known for its therapeutic properties is peppermint, which has a tradition in herbal medicine for soothing the digestive tract and relieving symptoms of digestive discomfort. And there appears to be some reasonable scientific evidence in support of using peppermint oil for irritable bowel syndrome, most likely owing to its antispasmodic properties.

But where there is evidence of this sort of benefit, it usually involves peppermint oil capsules. And I can't imagine you'd get anything like the concentrated dose of volatile oil from sipping on a home-made tea brewed from some freshly plucked mint leaves, but it tastes great and that's the whole point.

## How to buy it

When it comes to culinary uses, fresh is most definitely best. You can pick this up from pretty much any supermarket but it's totally easy to grow your own, too. In fact, a bit too easy, so unless you want your garden completely over-run with the stuff (I speak from experience), you're best off growing it in a large container or pot.

## How to cook it

If you've not made tea using fresh mint leaves before, then you've seriously got to give it a go. And there's a whole heap of other uses for mint, too. It's a total winner in a yoghurt dressing (in fact, I'd happily stick some fresh mint into the salad itself – think Tabbouleh). Not forgetting new potatoes and of course, minty mushy peas.

## Mint tea

A hot drink for a hot day. This is surprisingly refreshing.

For 4–6 cups

25 g (1 oz) fresh mint, leaves only
2 green tea teabags or 1 tbsp loose leaf
1 litre (2 pts) just boiled water
A light honey to taste

Take the mint leaves in your hands, reserving 4 of them for garnish, and crush gently so that the leaves break and start releasing their oils ■ Put the crushed leaves and green tea into a tea pot and pour over the just boiled water. Leave to brew for 3 minutes ■ Pour into small cups or heatproof glasses, garnish with a fresh mint leaf and serve immediately. A little honey can be added to sweeten if preferred.

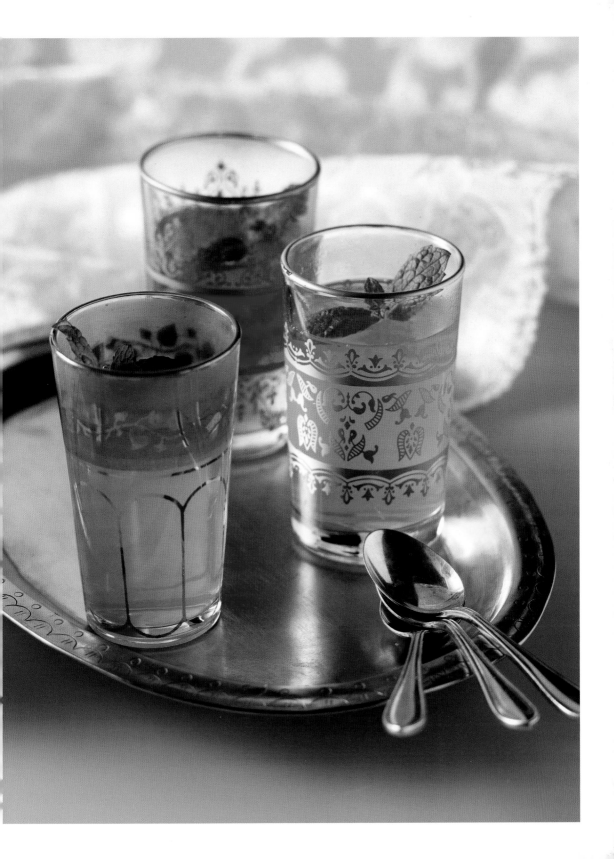

# The coffee shop

I've got this theory that we've all been brain-washed into thinking

that anything that tastes good and is enjoyable must definitely be bad

for us. At least, that's what the 'Food Police' would have us believe

anyway. What a load of tosh, I say.

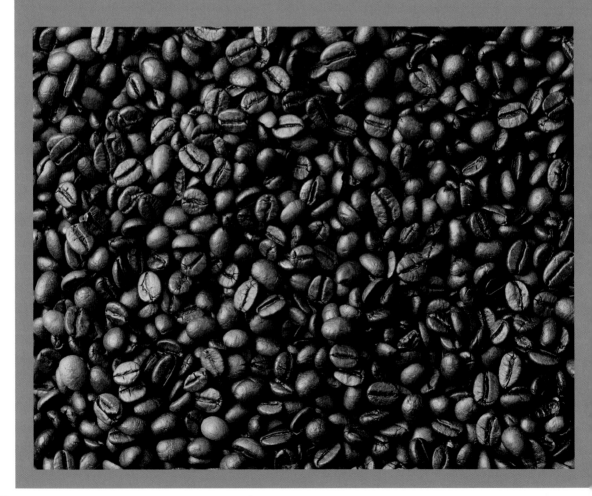

# Coffee

If I told you there was a drink that might reduce the risk of type II diabetes, Parkinson's disease, liver cirrhosis, gallstones and maybe even some cancers such as liver cancer, you'd probably be swigging it back with gusto. And you might be surprised to find out it's the nice-tasting, steaming black stuff they sell in Starbucks. As it happens, there's quite a lot of scientific research out there to support some of the potential health benefits of coffee drinking. But, before you stick the kettle on, it's important to realize that the type of evidence these findings are based on is mostly from population-based observational studies, and whilst of interest, can't prove cause and effect.

If we actually look at what's in coffee, we might be less surprised to see that it could quite feasibly qualify as a health beverage. Most folk tend to think that coffee = caffeine. But coffee is made up of many constituents other than just caffeine, packed with all sorts of phytochemicals. For example, it's a rich source of antioxidants, notably the polyphenol chlorogenic acid. Whilst we tend to think that antioxidants only come from blueberries, green tea or red wine, coffee appears to be a pretty significant source in our diets.

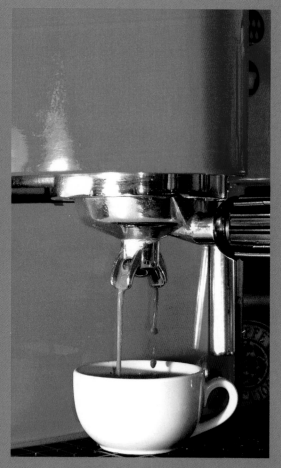

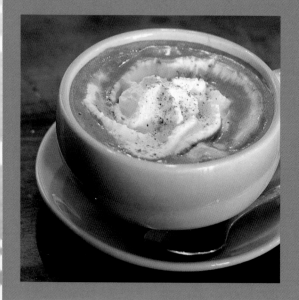

But before we get too carried away, coffee's not all good. Due to its relatively high caffeine content, some will find coffee the cause of nervousness, anxiety, even insomnia. Not to mention the possibility of withdrawal effects. It may also contribute to osteoporosis by increasing the amount of calcium excreted in the urine, raise blood pressure and raise levels of homocysteine, a risk factor for heart disease. And caffeine intake in pregnancy or whilst breastfeeding should certainly be strictly limited.

At the end of the day, coffee won't suit everybody. So if you don't like it or for whatever reason should be limiting or avoiding it, then steer clear of the stuff. But, if you can and do enjoy a coffee, chances are it will do you more good than harm.

## Black tea

Some of us tend to think of black tea as 'real' tea. Yet whilst super-slick green tea has stolen all the health plaudits, black tea has been left to stew. But despite a more drab image, black tea has got a lot going for it.

A bit like fruits and vegetables tea contains high levels of antioxidants, particularly a group of polyphenols known as flavonoids. And tea makes a substantial contribution to our dietary intake of flavonoids, especially in countries that are partial to a brew such as the UK.

Whilst green tea boasts more catechins (more of that in a minute), black tea contains more complex flavonoids by the names of theaflavins and thearubigins, generated when the leaves undergo oxidation in their production. Yet despite these differences, the antioxidant properties of black tea isn't far off the pace of green tea.

Black tea's main claim to fame is its association with a reduced risk of heart disease. And that's most likely down to its rich content of cardio-protective flavonoids.

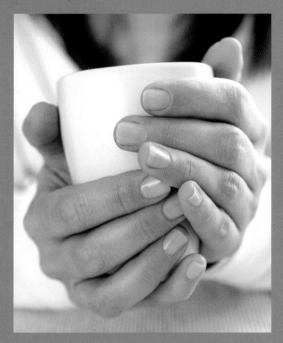

A common misconception I come across is that tea drinking contributes to bone loss and osteoporosis due to the negative effects of caffeine. Yet if anything, what evidence there is suggests the opposite, with regular consumption of tea appearing to protect bone density, especially in older women. And due to its high fluoride content, black tea could also theoretically help prevent tooth decay.

Another possible down-side to drinking tea is the effect of phenolic compounds on inhibiting iron absorption from food, potentially increasing the risk of anaemia. Consequently, those at risk of iron deficiency would be well advized to watch their intake and avoid drinking tea at mealtimes.

In terms of caffeine content, the average cup of tea weighs in with roughly a third to half the caffeine content of a typical cup of coffee. So whilst it's lower, individuals sensitive to caffeine or who need to moderate or avoid it for whatever reason, such as in pregnancy or due to specific health problems, should exercise due caution.

## Green tea

Compared with black tea, green tea contains much higher levels of catechins, the subject of a mountain of research, and the chief component likely to explain many of the brew's purported health benefits, such as a positive effect on cardiovascular health.

There's a whole bunch of interest in the potential cancer preventive effects of green tea, and in particular it's most abundant catechin, epigallocatechin gallate (or EGCG for short). Admittedly, a lot of the data comes from clever experiments done in test tubes or in animal studies, but there is also intriguing data from studies of human populations. Whilst the picture is far from complete and many uncertainties remain, the data suggests that consumption of green tea could potentially help to lower the risks of several types of cancer including breast and prostate.

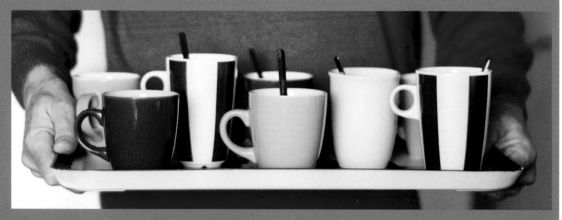

Green tea is also showing potential promise in a number of other areas such as in improving dental health and bolstering bone density, helping to protect against brain ageing and neurodegenerative disorders (such as Alzheimer's disease and Parkinson's disease), aiding in controlling body weight and even protecting the skin from the damaging effects of the sun.

Green tea weighs in with a lower caffeine content than black tea, although the same precautions apply.

## White tea

Just like black tea and green tea, white tea hails from the same tea plant, *Camellia sinensis*. It's basically akin to green tea in that it is unfermented and minimally processed. The big difference is that the leaves are picked before they're fully open, when they're still buds. And it's the fine silvery hairs that give the buds a distinctive white colour that gives rise to the tea's name. The taste is distinctively different to green tea, too, with less of the green grassy taste. Even my Dad, the last person on earth to drink 'herbal tea', likes it!

Due to its close similarity with green tea, the health benefits of white tea are likely to be pretty much comparable. Being the most minimally processed form of tea, there is some suggestion that white tea may be even higher in health promoting phytochemicals than green tea, although how this might translate to health benefits is not clear.

## Rooibos (Red Bush) tea

Unlike the good old fashioned cup of black tea that many of us are well accustomed to, rooibos tea has popped up practically out of nowhere and is giving our more traditional brew a run for its money. And meteoric has been its rise, making the transition from health food shop obscurity to glitzy supermarket-shelf stardom quicker than you can say, "put the kettle on".

Coming from the shrub *Aspalathus linearis*, rooibos is altogether different from traditional black or green tea derived from the *Camellia sinensis* plant. And one of the major differences is the fact that rooibos is naturally caffeine-free. A boon for anyone who doesn't tolerate caffeine well.

The potential health benefits of rooibos haven't been studied anywhere near as intensively as black or green tea, and many of its purported benefits remain the stuff of anecdote and folklore, not hard and fast scientific fact.

But to its credit, rooibos tea does appear to be a rich source of polyphenols, which show antioxidant properties and possible health benefits, so it may yet surprise us.

# Red wine

Whilst irresponsibly drinking a load of booze can have dire consequences for health, small amounts of alcohol can confer some health benefits.

Let's get to grips with the alcohol bit first. It looks likely that regular, modest amounts of alcohol are likely to protect against coronary heart disease in those at risk. It gets better. A modest consumption of alcohol is also associated with a decreased risk of type II diabetes. Good times.

Red wine has garnered particular interest due to the much touted 'French Paradox'. This refers to the fact that despite quaffing substantial amounts of saturated fat (steak frites, foie gras and lovely cheese) and puffing away on their fair share of fags, the French have surprisingly low rates of deaths from heart attacks. And this has been, at least in part, ascribed to their penchant for red wine and the high levels of polyphenolic compounds it contains. These beneficial antioxidant plant compounds are found in high concentrations within and just under the skin of red grapes and end up in the plonk.

The most hyped of these compounds is resveratrol, which has been shown to have cardio-protective properties. But most of this is stuff done in clever experiments, which doesn't always translate to what happens inside us humans. Ultimately how much of the cardiovascular benefits of red wine are down to these plant compounds, and how much is just an effect of the alcohol itself, is up for debate.

But it's not all sunshine and roses. When it comes to another major disease, cancer, the consensus of experts from across the globe is that there is no 'safe' intake of alcohol that is completely without risk.

Of course, it's about living in the real world and enjoying life to the full, and that means weighing up the pros and cons. On balance, that all points to what we know already, namely that our alcohol intake should definitely stick within safe recommended levels. That way we might reap the benefits, whilst minimizing the risks.

I know it's stating the obvious, but alcohol should be completely avoided by some groups such as children and during pregnancy, and in various health conditions or whilst taking certain medications. Common sense applies.

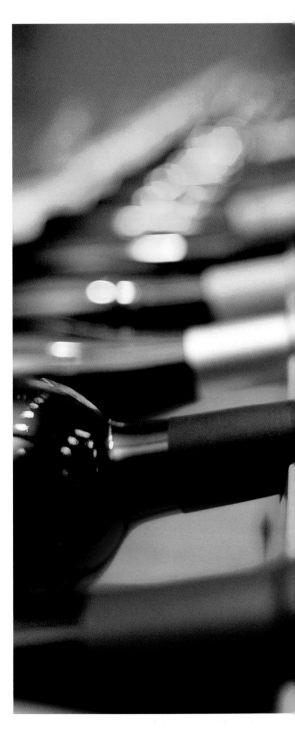

# Index

INDEX

INDEX

# Acknowledgements

The first and biggest thanks to Louise, for all her ace recipes and ideas and at least a million other things, and mostly just for being there and making sure this book got done. Massive thanks to Belle for developing loads of the great recipes that grace this book, a real talent in the making. Big thanks to mum for trying so many of the recipes and even managing to get dad to eat (and like) them. The legend that is Matt Hedges, I salute you and your taste buds. Diana and Sally (and the rest of the Hargrave family who no doubt tucked in!), what can I say? Thank you. The Sussex Uni old skool, Adam and Michael, cheers boys. My MSc buddies, Patsy and Kyla, a big thank you. Simon, the original curry fiend, cheers mate. A big thank you to Pat and Darren and their trusty taste buds. Not forgetting the forever youthful Louise Thomas-Minns. Thanks too to Debbie, and her lovely children Amy and Ben for their recipe road testing. A shout out to

Paul, Lucy, Betsy and Griff for getting stuck into the recipes. The inimitable Steve Howard, cheers mate. A big thanks to Gill (good to see you finally got some use out of the cooker!) and to Kev, for devouring everything I made, even the stuff that went wrong. Huge thanks too to the culinary skills of Benny and discerning tastes of young Frankie. Also to Colin for his ever valuable and enthusiastic feedback. And Lynn for the wicked quinoa recipe.

Borra and the good folk at DML, finally, I done it! Thanks for your support and guidance. Thanks to my editor Emma Pattison for all the hard work and help, and to Clare Sayer for totally clocking what this book was all about and getting it commissioned. Thanks to Sue Atkinson for all the great photography, and Eliza Baird for making the food look the business. And last but by no means least, the biggest dude of all, Jasper the cat, for hanging out with me the whole time.

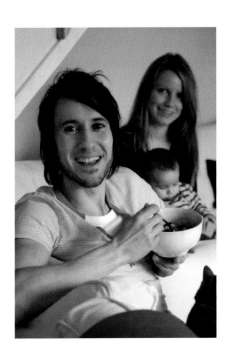

First published in 2009 by New Holland Publishers (UK) Ltd
London • Cape Town • Sydney • Auckland
www.newhollandpublishers.com

Garfield House • 86–88 Edgware Road • London W2 2EA • United Kingdom

80 McKenzie Street • Cape Town 8001 • South Africa

Unit 1, 66 Gibbes Street • Chatswood NSW 2067 • Australia

218 Lake Road • Northcote • Auckland • New Zealand

2 4 6 8 10 9 7 5 3 1

ISBN 978 1 84773 440 2

Publishing Director: **Rosemary Wilkinson**
Publisher: **Clare Sayer**
Senior Editor: **Emma Pattison**
Designer: **Fiona Andreanelli (www.andreanelli.com)**
Photographer: **Sue Atkinson**
Recipe Developer: **Belle Wiley**
Food Stylist: **Eliza Baird**
Props Stylist: **Roisin Nield**
Senior Production Controller: **Marion Storz**

Reproduction by Pica Digital Pte Ltd, Singapore
Printed and bound by Times Offset (M) Sdn Bhd, Malaysia

DISCLAIMER: This book should not be considered a replacement for professional medical
treatment; a physician should be consulted on all matters relating to health. While the information
in this book is believed to be accurate, neither the author nor the publisher can accept any legal
responsibility for any injury or illness sustained while following the given advice.